D0781411

Frye's
2500
Nursing
Bullets
NCLEX-PN

SECOND EDITION

Charles M. Frye, RN
Director
Professional Development Systems
School of Health Sciences
Long Beach, California

Springhouse Corporation
Springhouse, Pennsylvania

STAFF

Vice President
Matthew Cahill

Clinical Director
Judith A. Schilling McCann, RN, MSN

Art Director
John Hubbard

Managing Editor
David Moreau

Clinical Project Manager
Beverly Ann Tscheschlog, RN

Editors
Karen Diamond, Carol Munson

Copy Editors
Brenna H. Mayer (manager), Priscilla DeWitt, Jake Marcus-Cipolla, Jaime Stockslager, Pamela Wingrod

Designers
Arlene Putterman (associate art director), Donna S. Morris (project manager)

Manufacturing
Deborah Meiris (director), Patricia K. Dorshaw (manager), Otto Mezei (book production manager)

Editorial Assistants
Beverly Lane, Marcia Mills, Liz Schaeffer

Indexer
Kathy Wasong

The clinical procedures described and recommended in this publication are based on research and consultation with nursing, medical, and legal authorities. To the best of our knowledge, these procedures reflect currently accepted practice; nevertheless, they cannot be considered absolute and universal recommendations. For individual application, all recommendations must be considered in light of the patient's clinical condition and, before administration of new or infrequently used drugs, in light of the latest package-insert information. The author and the publisher disclaim responsibility for any adverse effects resulting directly or indirectly from the suggested procedures, from any undetected errors, or from the reader's misunderstanding of the text.

©2000 by Springhouse Corporation. All rights reserved. No part of this publication may be used or reproduced in any manner whatsoever without written permission except for brief quotations embodied in critical articles and reviews. For information, write Springhouse Corporation, 1111 Bethlehem Pike, P.O. Box 908, Springhouse, PA 19477-0908. Authorization to photocopy items for internal or personal use, or the internal or personal use of specific clients, is granted by Springhouse Corporation for users registered with the Copyright Clearance Center (CCC) Transactional Reporting Service, provided that the fee of $.75 per page is paid directly to CCC, 222 Rosewood Dr., Danvers, MA 01923. For those organizations that have been granted a photocopy license by CCC, a separate system of payment has been arranged. The fee code for users of the Transactional Reporting Service is 1582550077/2000 $00.00 + $.75.

Printed in the United States of America.

PNBTS2-D   N
02 01 00 99   10 9 8 7 6 5 4 3 2 1

℞ A member of the Reed Elsevier plc group

Library of Congress Cataloging-in-Publication Data

Frye, Charles M.
Frye's 2500 nursing bullets NCLEX-PN / Charles M. Frye. — 2nd ed.
    p. cm.
    Includes index.
    1. Practical nursing Examinations, questions, etc. 2. Practical nursing Outlines, syllabi, etc. I. Frye, Charles M. Frye's 2,000 nursing bullets NCLEX-PN. II. Title. III. Title: Frye's twenty-five hundred nursing bullets NCLEX-PN. IV. Title: 2,500 nursing bullets NCLEX-PN. [DNLM: 1. Nursing, Practical Examination Questions. WY 18.2F948f 1999]
RT62.F79 1999
610.73'076—dc21
DNLM/DLC   99-40688
ISBN 1-58255-007-7 (alk. paper)   CIP

To Cynthia Mapp (formerly of Lou's Book Store,
Long Beach, California), who helped me be "discovered"
by Jim Landis of Springhouse Corporation.
I am forever indebted to her.

Preface

In the more than 300 nursing review seminars that I have conducted, one thing is certain — when it comes to preparing for examinations, nursing candidates don't want to waste time learning things they don't need to know.

Unfortunately, no one knows with any certainty what will be on the next NCLEX-PN examination. Generally, candidates try to learn everything. They over-study certain areas, under-study others, and neglect the rest.

This is where *Frye's 2500 Nursing Bullets NCLEX-PN,* Second Edition, can make a difference. It's designed as a quick reference to numerous nursing procedures and disease processes, ideas on taking the NCLEX-PN, and tidbits of information that routinely surface on the examination.

This book is also ideal for nursing students; they can refer to it as they progress through their programs. It offers a condensed view of the nursing program packed into an easy-to-carry book.

How to use this book

Frye's 2500 Nursing Bullets NCLEX-PN, Second Edition, is designed to help you review for the NCLEX-PN effectively and efficiently. This book gives you nursing information that remains true in every clinical situation and setting, and these are the very facts that question writers must draw on in devising the test.

Follow these suggestions to get the most from this unique book:

▶ Read the introduction to prepare for computerized adaptive testing, learn about the NCLEX-PN test plan, and develop effective test-taking strategies.

▶ Study the key facts as they're presented in random order. You'll realize two benefits from this approach: You'll master essential data in psychiatric, pediatric, maternal, and medical-surgical nursing as well as the important concepts in nursing fundamentals, and you'll prepare yourself for the computerized NCLEX-PN, which also presents questions in a random style. (*Note:* After each bulleted fact in this book, the applicable clinical topic area appears in parentheses: FND for fundamentals, MAT for maternal-neonatal nursing, PED for pediatric nursing, M-S for medical-surgical nursing, and PSY for psychiatric nursing.)

▶ Review groups of nursing bullets throughout the day. Because this book is compact and easy to carry, you can take it with you wherever you go and review a few bullets whenever you have a spare minute — while waiting for class to begin, during a break between labs, or while riding the bus or train.

▶ Use the book to create questions to quiz your study partner or members of your study group.

No matter how you choose to use this versatile book, you'll find that each nursing bullet is brief, easy to read, and free from distracting clinical situations and excess wording. You'll find that you'll easily remember and identify the facts, no matter what form they take on the test. Because each bullet has been reviewed by a clinical expert, you can be sure that all the information is up-to-date and clinically accurate.

You've spent years studying to become a nurse and months preparing for the NCLEX-PN. Now, with *Frye's 2500 Nursing Bullets NCLEX-PN*, Second Edition, you can take this last step to licensure with confidence.

Introduction

In the United States, if you want to work as a licensed practical nurse, you need a license from the nursing licensure authority in the state where you plan to practice. To get a license, you need to pass the National Council Licensure Examination for Practical Nurses (NCLEX-PN). This book will help you do just that. Its 2,500 bullets of nursing facts will expand and reinforce your nursing knowledge base. Further, this introduction will prepare you for the examination by describing the new computerized adaptive testing system, explaining the NCLEX-PN test plan, and providing effective test-taking strategies.

Scheduling your test

To schedule your NCLEX-PN examination, apply to your state board of nursing for testing. When your application is approved, the Educational Testing Service Data Center will send you an Authorization to Test and will advise you to make an examination appointment at one of 200 Sylvan Technology Centers throughout the country.

When scheduling your NCLEX-PN, remember that the test takes up to 5 hours and is offered 15 hours daily, Monday through Saturday, and sometimes on Sunday. The Sylvan Technology Center will schedule you for testing within 30 days of your call (or within 45 days for retesting). If you need to reschedule your examination appointment, call the Sylvan Technology Center at least 3 days beforehand.

Understanding computerized adaptive testing

Since April of 1994, the NCLEX-PN has been a computerized test. It requires you to answer a sufficient number of questions at various levels of difficulty to demonstrate minimum competence as an entry-level nurse. It's adaptive because it selects harder or easier questions based on your response to previous questions. For example, if you answer a medium-level question correctly, the computer will pose a more difficult question next. If you answer incorrectly, it will choose an easier one.

The test bank includes thousands of questions categorized by level of difficulty and the NCLEX-PN test plan. From this bank, the computer continues to pull questions until you demonstrate competence in all parts of the test plan. Therefore, each test is different and may require 85 to 205 questions to complete.

Before the test, a proctor will help you get started at a computer terminal. The test will begin with brief instructions and a practice session of 15 questions. During the practice session and the test, use only the space bar (to move the cursor to the four answer options) and the enter key (to select your answer). To avoid unintentional answers, the computer will ask you to confirm your answer selection by striking the enter key again.

During the test, the computer will display one question at a time. If a case study is included, it will appear to the left of the question. Consider each question carefully. Then press the space bar to move to the option that best answers the question. To record your answer, press the enter key twice. Because the computer doesn't let you skip questions or return to previous items, you must answer every question until the test ends.

The testing period includes a mandatory 10-minute break after 2 hours and an optional break 90 minutes after testing resumes.

Understanding the NCLEX-PN test plan

The NCLEX-PN test plan classifies questions by the five steps of the nursing process and the four categories of client needs. Each test question reflects one nursing process step and one client needs category.

Nursing process steps

The nursing process is a five-step method of performing nursing care. On the NCLEX-PN test, each nursing process step carries equal weight.

▶ *Data collection* refers to forming a database by gathering subjective and objective information about a patient.

▶ *Analysis,* or nursing diagnosis, refers to identifying actual or potential health problems based on assessment findings.

▶ *Planning* refers to establishing goals to meet the patient's needs and developing strategies for achieving those goals.

▶ *Implementation* refers to performing actions that accomplish the patient's established goals.

▶ *Evaluation* refers to measuring the extent of goal achievement.

Client needs

The health needs of patients are organized by four major categories of client needs. These were identified during a 1997 job analysis study of newly licensed practical nurses. They consist of four categories and 10 subcategories, which are:

A. Safe, effective care environment

1. Coordinated care (6% to 12%)
▶ Providing integrated, cost-effective care to patients by coordinating, supervising, or collaborating with members of the multidisciplinary health care team

2. Safety and infection control (7% to 13%)
▶ Protecting patients and health care personnel from environmental hazards

B. Health promotion and maintenance

1. Growth and development through the life span (4% to 10%)
▶ Assisting patients and significant others through the normal expected stages of growth and development from conception through advanced old age

2. Prevention and early detection of disease (4% to 10%)
▶ Managing and providing care for patients in need of prevention and early detection of health problems

C. Psychosocial integrity

1. Coping and adaptation (6% to 12%)
▶ Promoting the ability of patients to cope, adapt, or troubleshoot situations related to illnesses or stressful events

2. Psychosocial adaptation (4% to 10%)
▶ Managing and providing care for patients with acute or chronic mental illnesses

D. Physiological integrity

1. Basic care and comfort (10% to 16%)
▶ Providing comfort and assistance in the performance of activities of daily living

2. Pharmacological therapies (5% to 11%)
▶ Managing and providing care related to the administration of medications

3. Reduction of risk potential (11% to 17%)
► Reducing the likelihood that patients will develop complications or health problems related to existing conditions, treatments, or procedures

4. Physiological adaptation (13% to 19%)
► Managing and providing care to patients with acute, chronic, or life-threatening physical health conditions

Studying for the examination

To study for the NCLEX-PN as effectively as possible and enhance your ability to retain pertinent information, follow these study tips:

► Familiarize yourself with all examination topics.

► Answer as many practice questions as possible. (You may want to use this book's bullets to develop study questions with a partner.)

► Understand the parts of a test question. On the NCLEX-PN, each multiple-choice question has a stem (the question itself) and four options: a key (correct answer) and three distracters (incorrect answers). A brief case study may precede any question.

► Use additional study guides as resources, such as the *American Nursing Review for NCLEX-PN,* if desired.

► Organize a study group with other nursing students or take an NCLEX review course.

► Ask a colleague or nursing instructor to clarify unfamiliar or complex material.

Planning for the examination

Remember that the NCLEX-PN poses certain physical demands. To cope with these demands, ensure your best test performance, and help you plan for the examination, use these pointers:

► Schedule your test appointment at a testing center near your home, if possible. Before the test, assess the parking facilities and determine travel time.

► Make reservations well in advance at a hotel near the testing center if you must travel a long distance.

▶ Schedule your test appointment to take advantage of your peak-performance time.

▶ Avoid late-night, last-minute cramming. Obtain sufficient sleep the night before the test.

▶ Eat a well-balanced meal before the test.

▶ Wear layers of clothes that can be removed, as needed, to maintain warmth and comfort.

▶ Take your Authorization to Test and two forms of identification with signatures (including one photographic identification) to the testing center. You can't take the examination without them.

▶ Use simple relaxation techniques, such as progressive relaxation, during the test to reduce anxiety.

Developing test-taking skills

Knowing the facts isn't all you need to pass the NCLEX-PN. You also need to know how to take the test. To sharpen your test-taking skills, review these guidelines:

▶ Check case studies closely for information needed to answer the question correctly.

▶ Look for clue words, such as *best*, *first*, *most*, and *not* in the question's stem. These words, which may be highlighted, aid in selecting the correct answer.

▶ Imagine the correct response when reading the stem. If it appears as one of the four options, it's probably the correct one.

▶ Read every question and all four of its options carefully before making your final selection.

▶ Reread the stem and options when two options seem equally correct; look again for clues or differences that can help you select the correct answer. When in doubt, make an educated guess. Remember: You can't skip questions.

▶ Don't panic if a question covers an unfamiliar topic. Draw on your knowledge of similar problems and nursing principles to help eliminate options and increase the chance of choosing the correct answer.

▶ Take your time and pace yourself. Don't spend excessive time on any one question.

▶ Don't be distracted by other candidates or the apparent length of their tests. Keep in mind that each test is individualized.

▶ Use break periods to rest your mind and body — for example, eat a small snack, stretch, or do relaxation exercises.

Frye's
2500
Nursing
Bullets

NCLEX-PN

SECOND EDITION

▶ When a closed water-seal chest drainage system is attached properly to suction, fluctuation occurs in the water-seal chamber. **(M-S)**

▶ During a liver biopsy, the nurse should instruct the patient to hold his breath, turn his head to the left, and place his right hand under his head while the needle is inserted. **(M-S)**

▶ After the patient has a liver biopsy, the nurse should position the patient on the right side with a pillow under the liver border. **(M-S)**

▶ After the patient has a pneumonectomy, the nurse promotes full expansion of the patient's unaffected lung by helping the patient ambulate, perform incentive spirometry, and lie on the affected side. **(M-S)**

▶ When collecting a 24-hour urine specimen, discard the first voiding and begin the 24-hour collection with the next specimen. **(M-S)**

▶ The frequency of labor contractions is assessed by timing from the beginning of one contraction to the beginning of the next and is measured in minutes. **(MAT)**

▶ The duration of labor contractions is assessed by timing from the start to the end of uterine muscle contraction and is measured in seconds. **(MAT)**

▶ For the patient with epiglottitis, the nurse should keep a tracheostomy set at the bedside for immediate use in case of airway obstruction. **(M-S)**

▶ Spills of blood should be cleaned up with a fresh 1:10 solution of sodium hypochlorite (household bleach) in water. **(M-S)**

▶ If a child has recurrent otitis media, the nurse should ask the parents about compliance with prescribed drug therapy. **(PED)**

▶ To prevent hip flexion contractures following a leg amputation, avoid placing the residual limb on pillows and elevating the head of the bed higher than 60 degrees. Turn patient prone twice a day. **(M-S)**

▶ Ritualistic behavior is any repetitive act performed by the patient with obsessive-compulsive disorder. **(PSY)**

▶ The best method for preventing nosocomial infections is washing hands between patient contacts. **(M-S)**

▶ The patient with an amputation may experience phantom sensation or pain. **(M-S)**

▶ The nurse can acquire a nosocomial infection while carrying out usual nursing duties. **(M-S)**

▶ After the nurse has contact with a patient who is considered uncontaminated, hand washing for 15 to 30 seconds is generally considered sufficient for infection control. **(FND)**

▶ Mannitol (Osmitrol), a hypertonic solution, is used to treat patients with cerebral edema. **(M-S)**

▶ During mannitol therapy, the patient should have an indwelling urinary catheter so that urine output can be accurately monitored. **(M-S)**

▶ Rocky Mountain spotted fever is transmitted through the bite of a tick. **(M-S)**

▶ If a child is suspected of having epiglottitis or croup, the nurse shouldn't examine the inside of the child's throat or take an oral temperature. **(PED)**

▶ A characteristic sign of Lyme disease is an expanding bull's eye erythematous lesion that may appear anywhere on the body. **(M-S)**

▶ Giardiasis is a protozoal infection of the small intestine that causes protracted diarrhea. **(M-S)**

▶ During two-person cardiopulmonary resuscitation, the rescuers perform five chest compressions to one ventilation. **(M-S)**

▶ During one-person cardiopulmonary resuscitation, the rescuer performs fifteen chest compressions to two ventilations. **(M-S)**

▶ The organization that formulates nursing diagnoses is the North American Nursing Diagnosis Association. **(FND)**

▶ Signs of fetal alcohol syndrome generally present within the first 24 hours of life. **(MAT)**

▶ An adverse effect of digoxin is nausea. **(M-S)**

▶ Following circumcision, the infant should be closely monitored for bleeding. **(MAT)**

▶ Cervical dilation occurs in an inevitable abortion, but not in a threatened abortion. **(MAT)**

▶ Two medications used to treat Parkinson's disease include levodopa (Dopar) and carbidopa-levodopa (Sinemet). **(M-S)**

▶ Five types of hallucinations exist: visual, auditory, tactile, gustatory, and olfactory. **(PSY)**

▶ For the patient with a Sengstaken-Blakemore tube, the nurse should keep a pair of scissors at the bedside for emergency deflation. **(M-S)**

▶ The fat-soluble vitamins are A, D, E, and K. **(M-S)**

▶ Starch is the most abundant dietary carbohydrate. **(M-S)**

▶ The nurse should assess for dependent edema in the lower extremities, such as the ankles (in a dependent position) in the ambulatory patient or the sacrum in the wheelchair-bound patient. **(M-S)**

▶ In an autograft, the patient's own skin is taken from one site and transplanted to another site. **(M-S)**

▶ In a homograft, skin is taken from a cadaver 6 to 24 hours after death and transplanted to an individual of the same species. **(M-S)**

▶ The characteristic sign of primary syphilis is a painless, fluid-filled lesion called a chancre. **(M-S)**

▶ Many women with gonorrhea have no signs or symptoms of this sexually transmitted disease. **(M-S)**

▶ Ménière's disease produces a triad of symptoms: vertigo, hearing loss, and tinnitus. **(M-S)**

▶ Vitamin C promotes wound healing. **(M-S)**

▶ To decrease the risk of urinary tract infection, the patient should wash the perineal area with soap and water twice a day and after each bowel movement. **(M-S)**

▶ A smooth, sore, red, beefy tongue is a sign of pernicious anemia. **(M-S)**

▶ A major concern for the patient receiving total parenteral nutrition is the risk of hyperglycemia. **(M-S)**

▶ To prevent hypoglycemia when total parenteral nutrition is being discontinued, the nurse should gradually taper off the amount administered, as ordered, and provide the patient with oral carbohydrates. These actions allow the body to adjust to the decreasing glucose level. **(M-S)**

▶ To administer a routine cleansing enema effectively, the nurse should place the adult patient on his left side. **(M-S)**

▶ The normal arterial blood pH ranges from 7.35 to 7.45. **(FND)**

▶ Split-thickness grafts, which include two upper layers of skin (epidermis) and part of the middle layer (dermis), are used frequently in early stages of burns. **(M-S)**

▶ In skin grafts, a heat lamp is used to dry the donor site, promote epithelization from deeper layers of skin, and prevent infection. **(M-S)**

▶ During heparin (Liquaemin) therapy, the patient should receive acetaminophen (Tylenol) for headaches, not aspirin. **(M-S)**

▶ The preferred I.M. injection site for a small child is the vastus lateralis muscle. **(FND)**

▶ When trying to understand how a patient feels about a disturbing issue, the nurse uses empathy. **(PSY)**

▶ Signs of lithium carbonate toxicity include diarrhea, vomiting, drowsiness, muscle weakness, and ataxia. **(PSY)**

▶ A milliequivalent (mEq) is the unit of measurement used to describe the chemical activity of electrolytes; mEq is the number of milligrams per 100 milliliters of a solution. **(FND)**

▶ When the patient checks out of the hospital against the doctor's advice, documentation should indicate that the patient left AMA (against medical advice). **(FND)**

▶ Dietary fiber can't be digested by human enzymes and can't be absorbed from the small intestine. **(M-S)**

▶ To prevent dorsiflexion of the foot, and footdrop, in the patient who is immobilized, a footboard should be provided. **(M-S)**

▶ In chronic venous insufficiency, the body develops collateral blood flow to the affected area. **(M-S)**

▶ In acute venous insufficiency, collateral blood flow doesn't have an opportunity to develop. **(M-S)**

▶ Following a cerebrovascular accident, motor impulses usually return in 2 to 14 days. **(M-S)**

▶ Oxytocin (Pitocin) is administered to promote uterine contractions. **(MAT)**

▶ During the latent phase of the first stage of labor, the patient's cervix dilates from 0 to 4 cm. **(MAT)**

▶ During the active phase of the first stage of labor, the patient's cervix dilates from 4 to 8 cm. **(MAT)**

▶ During the transitional phase of the first stage of labor, the patient's cervix dilates from 8 to 10 cm. **(MAT)**

▶ During the first stage of labor, effacement becomes complete, and expulsion of the neonate begins. **(MAT)**

▶ The second stage of labor begins with complete cervical effacement and dilation, and ends with delivery of the fetus. **(MAT)**

▶ The third stage of labor begins after the birth of the neonate and ends with the delivery of the placenta. **(MAT)**

▶ The fourth stage of labor begins with expulsion of the placenta and ends with postpartum stabilization **(MAT)**.

▶ Pulse pressure is the difference between the systolic and diastolic pressures (that is, if blood presure is 120/80, pulse pressure equals 40 mm Hg). **(M-S)**

▶ A pulse deficit refers to the difference between the apical pulse and a peripheral pulse, such as the radial pulse. **(FND)**

▶ The nurse should weigh the patient at the same time every day, using the same scale and with the patient wearing the same type of clothing. **(FND)**

▶ If the patient reports cramping during colostomy irrigation, the nurse should lower the bag to slow the flow rate. **(M-S)**

▶ The nurse should turn the neonate frequently during phototherapy and keep him hydrated. **(MAT)**

▶ The three phases of a uterine contraction are increment, decrement, and acme. **(MAT)**

▶ A febrile reaction is the most common transfusion reaction. **(M-S)**

▶ If jaundice is suspected in the neonate, the nurse should examine him under natural light or a white fluorescent light. **(MAT)**

▶ If the bottle-fed neonate doesn't begin to suck, the nurse should show the mother how to elicit the rooting reflex. **(MAT)**

▶ The first sign of bladder cancer is usually painless hematuria. **(M-S)**

▶ Before engaging in any strenuous activity, the patient with angina pectoris should take a nitroglycerin (Nitro-Bid) tablet. **(M-S)**

▶ The patient with pernicious anemia must take vitamin B_{12} injections for the remainder of his life. **(M-S)**

▶ The stress of hospitalization can precipitate a sickle cell crisis. **(M-S)**

▶ Maternal stress can decrease the breast milk supply. **(MAT)**

▶ Before administering an iron dextran (InFed) injection, the nurse should change the needle on the syringe. **(M-S)**

▶ To prevent tooth staining, the child should use a straw to drink a liquid iron preparation. **(PED)**

▶ Annual rectal examinations aid in early detection of prostate cancer. **(M-S)**

▶ A sign of breast cancer is a nontender, nonmovable lump (usually in the upper outer quadrant). **(M-S)**

▶ The patient with orthopnea must sit or stand to breathe deeply or comfortably. **(M-S)**

▶ A positive Homans' sign (calf pain on dorsiflexion of the foot) is a sign of deep vein thrombosis. **(M-S)**

▶ The antidote for heparin is protamine sulfate. **(M-S)**

▶ Independent nursing actions are actions that the nurse initiates and has the requisite skills and knowledge to carry out. **(FND)**

▶ Subjective data is information supplied by the patient, a family member, or another health care provider that is based on opinion. **(FND)**

▶ Objective data is observable or measurable information. **(FND)**

▶ During the first 8 weeks after conception (the period of organogenesis), all organs are developed in a rudimentary form and the fetus is most susceptible to a teratogenic effect. **(MAT)**

▶ Signs of inflammation include pain, erythema, swelling, warmth, and loss of motor function. **(M-S)**

▶ A circadian rhythm is a cycle that repeats about once a day (24 hours). **(FND)**

▶ When performing passive range-of-motion exercises, don't force the extremity beyond the point of pain or continuous spasm. **(FND)**

▶ To shave the patient, the nurse should hold the razor at a 45-degree angle and use firm strokes in the direction of hair growth. **(FND)**

▶ A clove hitch is the best knot to secure a limb restraint because it won't tighten when pulled. **(FND)**

► The nurse should place a crib net over the crib to prevent the child under age 2 from climbing out. **(PED)**

► The pregnant teenager should be encouraged to select food high in iron and protein. **(MAT)**

► Canned or processed foods are high in sodium and should be restricted in patients with heart failure. **(M-S)**

► Give vitamin B and fat-soluble vitamins (A, D, E, K) to the patient with Laënnec's cirrhosis. **(M-S)**

► The scope is confined in a direct interview and the patient is asked only specific questions. **(FND)**

► During furosemide (Lasix) therapy, the patient is at risk for potassium loss, which can lead to hypokalemia. **(M-S)**

► Before obtaining a throat culture, the nurse should have the patient rinse his mouth with water. **(M-S)**

► Before providing a sputum sample, the patient shouldn't brush his teeth or use mouthwash. **(M-S)**

► Food eaten by the Orthodox Jewish patient must be kosher. **(FND)**

► A sign of fecal impaction is seepage of liquid stool. **(M-S)**

► The stools of a breast-fed infant are golden yellow, smooth, and pasty. **(PED)**

► Meconium is thick and usually green to black. **(MAT)**

► In a dark-skinned patient, the nurse should assess for petechiae on the oral mucosa, rather than the skin. **(M-S)**

► A woman with Rh-negative blood should receive an injection of $Rh_o(D)$ immune globulin (RhoGAM) within 72 hours after giving birth to a neonate with Rh-positive blood. **(MAT)**

► After birth, the nurse should suction the neonate's mouth immediately and then the nose. **(MAT)**

► When suctioning a tracheostomy, the nurse should apply suction as the catheter is being withdrawn from the trachea and should limit the number of passes in and out of the trachea to two. **(M-S)**

► A patient can hyperventilate by breathing too quickly or by breathing too deeply at a normal rate. **(M-S)**

▶ A patient can hypoventilate by breathing too slowly or by breathing too shallowly at a normal rate; the treatment is controlled breathing or having the patient breath into a paper bag. **(M-S)**

▶ For the mother who plans to breast-feed, the nurse should instruct her to "toughen" her nipples by rolling them between thumb and forefinger or rubbing them with a towel. **(MAT)**

▶ The mother who plans to breast-feed should be permitted to do so shortly after delivery. **(MAT)**

▶ A probable sign of pregnancy is a positive human chorionic gonadotropin value in blood or urine. **(MAT)**

▶ Positive signs of pregnancy include fetal presence on ultrasound, palpable fetal movement, and fetal heart tones. **(MAT)**

▶ Presumptive signs of pregnancy may include nausea, vomiting, and breast tenderness. **(MAT)**

▶ Gravidity refers to the total number of times the woman has been pregnant without reference to the outcome of the pregnancy. **(MAT)**

▶ Parity refers to the number of pregnancies that reached viability (20 weeks) regardless of whether the fetus was born alive. **(MAT)**

▶ For a 5-year-old child, one of the greatest fears about being hospitalized is the fear of mutilation. **(PED)**

▶ Weight gain after peritoneal dialysis indicates fluid retention and should be reported immediately to the unit manager. **(M-S)**

▶ Theophylline toxicity occurs when the serum theophylline level rises above 20 µg/ml. **(M-S)**

▶ Battered-child syndrome is one of the leading causes of childhood death and disability. **(PED)**

▶ When administering an antacid with cimetidine (Tagamet), the nurse should give the antacid 1 hour before the cimetidine. **(M-S)**

▶ After collecting a stool sample for ova and parasite testing, the nurse should send the sample immediately (while warm) to the laboratory. **(M-S)**

▶ A wound that heals with granulation is healing by secondary intention. **(M-S)**

▶ An ominous sign of increased intracranial pressure is widening pulse pressure. **(M-S)**

▶ A clinical sign of placenta previa is painless vaginal bleeding. **(MAT)**

▶ Fat provides 9 cal/g. **(FND)**

▶ Biological death occurs with the irreversible destruction and death of brain tissue. **(FND)**

▶ The nurse should use sterile technique when administering an I.M. injection. **(FND)**

▶ For the patient who is immobilized, the nurse should perform passive or active range-of-motion exercises at least twice daily. **(FND)**

▶ When performing range-of-motion exercises, the nurse should stop the exercise at the point the patient begins to feel pain. **(FND)**

▶ Respiratory insufficiency is the most common complication after pneumonectomy. **(M-S)**

▶ The cuff of gloves should be brought over gown sleeves. **(FND)**

▶ Medicare is a government-funded program that provides medical and hospital insurance to people age 65 and older. **(FND)**

▶ In Freud's phallic stage, the male child develops an Oedipus complex and the female child develops an Electra complex. **(PSY)**

▶ If liquid passes through a porous sterile field, the field is then considered unsterile. **(M-S)**

▶ Sordes is mucus accumulation and crust formation on the teeth and lips. **(M-S)**

▶ The patient in a cast can maintain muscle mass and strength by performing isometric exercises. **(FND)**

▶ According to Maslow's hierarchy of need, physiologic needs must be met before other needs can be addressed. **(FND)**

▶ During evaluation, the nurse determines if the patient goals have been met. **(FND)**

▶ Linea nigra is a dark line from the umbilicus to the mons pubis. **(MAT)**

▶ Implantation of the ovum occurs 7 to 10 days after fertilization. **(MAT)**

▶ For the first 24 hours after leg amputation, the foot of the bed should be raised to elevate the stump and prevent edema. **(M-S)**

▶ Lung cancer is the leading cause of cancer-related deaths among men in the United States. **(M-S)**

▶ Level of consciousness deteriorates in this order: alertness, lethargy, stupor, light coma, and deep coma. **(M-S)**

▶ Parkinson's disease is a progressive neurologic disease. **(M-S)**

▶ Generalized tonic-clonic seizures involve both hemispheres of the brain and cause both sides of the body to react. **(M-S)**

▶ Generalized tonic-clonic seizures usually are preceded by an aura. **(M-S)**

▶ Status epilepticus causes acute prolonged seizure activity with failure to regain consciousness between seizures. **(M-S)**

▶ The ideal donor for the patient who needs a kidney transplant is an identical twin sibling. **(M-S)**

▶ Lung cancer is the most common cancer in American women. **(M-S)**

▶ Curling's ulcer is a peptic or duodenal ulcer that results from severe stress associated with a serious burn. **(M-S)**

▶ One way to determine and record blood loss after a hysterectomy is to count the number of perineal pads used; saturating a pad an hour or ten pads in 24 hours is considered hemorrhaging. **(MAT)**

▶ The most common surgical treatment for benign prostatic hyperplasia is transurethral resection of the prostate. **(M-S)**

▶ With a chest tube attached to a drainage system, inhalation causes the water level in the water-seal chamber to move up. **(M-S)**

▶ Spinal fusion is used to stabilize the spine. **(M-S)**

▶ To logroll the patient, the nurse can use a draw sheet or obtain help from one or more nurses. **(M-S)**

▶ In placenta previa, abnormal implantation in the lower uterine segment causes the placenta to partially or completely cover the internal cervical os. **(MAT)**

▶ In central (total) placenta previa, the placenta completely covers the cervical os. **(MAT)**

▶ In partial (incomplete) placenta previa, the placenta covers only a portion of the cervical os. **(MAT)**

▶ In marginal (lateral) placenta previa, the placenta covers one side of the cervical os. **(MAT)**

▶ In abruptio placentae, a normally implanted placenta undergoes premature separation from the uterine wall. **(MAT)**

▶ Cutis marmorata is a transient vasomotor response that occurs primarily in the extremities of infants exposed to cold.   **(PED)**

▶ Eclampsia is pregnancy-induced hypertension.   **(MAT)**

▶ Mental retardation has four classifications: mild, moderate, severe, and profound.   **(M-S)**

▶ For the male patient who has reached puberty, the major complication of mumps is orchitis, which can lead to sterility.   **(M-S)**

▶ In women, a common complication of gonorrhea is pelvic inflammatory disease.   **(MAT)**

▶ In Hirschsprung's disease (congenital megacolon), a lack of peristalsis leads to abdominal distention.   **(M-S)**

▶ Scoliosis refers to a lateral S-shaped spinal curvature.   **(M-S)**

▶ According to Freud, infants are in the oral stage of psychosexual development.   **(PSY)**

▶ A sign of the secondary stage of syphilis may include a rash on the palms of the hands and soles of the feet.   **(M-S)**

▶ Alcoholics Anonymous uses a 12-step program to achieve sobriety; however, an alcoholic is never considered cured.   **(PSY)**

▶ For the patient receiving total parenteral nutrition, the nurse should monitor the glucose and electrolyte levels frequently.   **(M-S)**

▶ When treating substance abuse, the nurse should recognize that up to 90% of substance abusers will have relapses.   **(PSY)**

▶ When taken together, alcohol and barbiturates have an additive effect leading to severe central nervous system depression.   **(M-S)**

▶ A lithium level above 2 mEq/L is toxic.   **(PSY)**

▶ The patient taking a monoamine oxidase inhibitor should avoid tyramine-rich foods, such as aged cheese, chocolate, and monosodium glutamate.   **(PSY)**

▶ The nurse should use the bell of the stethoscope to hear low-pitched sounds such as heart murmurs.   **(FND)**

▶ A severe complication of a fractured femur is excessive blood loss, which can result in shock and renal failure.   **(M-S)**

▶ To prepare for peritoneal dialysis, a catheter is inserted through the abdominal wall into the peritoneal space.   **(M-S)**

▶ If more than 3 L of dialysate solution is returned during peritoneal dialysis, the nurse should notify the doctor. **(M-S)**

▶ Hemodialysis removes nitrogenous wastes and excess water from the blood. **(M-S)**

▶ In hemodialysis, wastes diffuse through a semipermeable membrane into the dialysate; water enters the dialysate by osmosis. **(M-S)**

▶ Kaposi's sarcoma is an opportunistic disease associated with acquired immunodeficiency syndrome. **(M-S)**

▶ Gangrene usually affects the digits first. **(M-S)**

▶ The nurse should use the diaphragm of the stethoscope to hear high-pitched sounds such as breath sounds. **(FND)**

▶ The blood pressure measurement commonly varies 5 to 10 mm Hg from one arm to the other; this difference is normal. **(FND)**

▶ The blood pressure cuff should cover about one-third of the patient's upper arm. **(FND)**

▶ To assess an obese patient's blood pressure, the nurse may need to use a thigh cuff and listen for heart sounds in the popliteal space. **(FND)**

▶ A blood pressure cuff that is too loose will yield too high a blood pressure reading. **(FND)**

▶ Ptosis is drooping of the eyelids. **(FND)**

▶ Overflow incontinence is characterized by frequent loss of urine from the bladder. **(M-S)**

▶ The nurse should perform a weight-bearing transfer only with a patient who has at least one strong leg. **(FND)**

▶ The first sign of a pressure ulcer is skin redness that blanches under pressure. **(M-S)**

▶ A tilt table allows gradual movement from a horizontal to a vertical position. **(FND)**

▶ Using a tilt table allows the patient's body to compensate for position changes. **(FND)**

▶ Sickle cell anemia involves a defect in the hemoglobin. **(M-S)**

▶ When measuring for crutches, the nurse should have the patient wear the shoes that he will use for walking. **(FND)**

▶ If a patient has taken oral contraceptives exactly as prescribed, she should continue taking them even if she misses her menstrual period.   **(M-S)**

▶ If a patient misses two consecutive menstrual periods while taking oral contraceptives as prescribed, she should stop taking the pills, notify her doctor, and have a pregnancy test.   **(M-S)**

▶ If a patient misses taking one oral contraceptive tablet, she should take it as soon as she remembers (or should take two at the next scheduled interval) and continue with the usual schedule.   **(M-S)**

▶ If a patient misses taking an oral contraceptive for two consecutive days, she should take two tablets each day for two days, resume the usual schedule, and use an additional contraceptive method for 1 week.   **(M-S)**

▶ Mechanical ventilation can maintain ventilation automatically for an extended time.   **(M-S)**

▶ Mechanical ventilation may be performed by a negative or positive pressure ventilator.   **(M-S)**

▶ Stable angina pectoris is characterized by substernal pain that is caused by myocardial ischemia and lasts 2 to 3 minutes.   **(M-S)**

▶ Angina pain that lasts for more than 20 minutes and isn't relieved by nitroglycerin indicates a developing myocardial infarction.   **(M-S)**

▶ A nitroglycerin test is positive if nitroglycerin administration relieves angina pain.   **(M-S)**

▶ The goal of treatment for the patient with angina pectoris is to reduce the heart's workload.   **(M-S)**

▶ Nitroglycerin causes generalized vasodilation, which promotes blood flow to the heart muscle.   **(M-S)**

▶ The nurse should teach the patient with angina who is receiving sublingual nitroglycerin (Nitro-Bid) to place a tablet under the tongue at the first sign of chest pain.   **(M-S)**

▶ The patient may repeat the nitroglycerin dosage every 5 to 15 minutes for a maximum of three tablets.   **(M-S)**

▶ If chest pain persists for more than 15 minutes, the patient should be instructed to go to the nearest health care facility.   **(M-S)**

▶ Hemodialysis may be performed 24 hours before a kidney transplant to remove accumulated waste products from the blood. **(M-S)**

▶ After a radical mastectomy, the patient's arm on the affected side may swell because the procedure removes lymph nodes and lymph vessels. **(M-S)**

▶ The patient who has had a radical mastectomy shouldn't have blood drawn from the affected arm. **(M-S)**

▶ In placenta previa, bleeding is painless, rarely fatal, and usually subsides spontaneously with the initial episode. **(MAT)**

▶ The patient who has had a mastectomy is prone to lymphedema. **(M-S)**

▶ Usually, the treatment for abruptio placentae is immediate delivery by cesarean section. **(MAT)**

▶ Nurses should transport hospitalized infants or children in strollers, wheelchairs, or beds — not in their arms. **(M-S)**

▶ When a protective device is used to restrain the patient, the nurse should attach it to the bed frame or to springs that move with the patient's head. **(M-S)**

▶ Signs of theophylline toxicity include vomiting, agitation, and an apical pulse above 200 beats/minute. **(M-S)**

▶ When teaching the parents of a child with croup, the nurse should instruct them not to administer cough syrup. **(PED)**

▶ The nurse shouldn't induce vomiting in the patient who has ingested poison and is semiconscious, comatose, or experiencing seizures. **(M-S)**

▶ The nurse is required to report all suspected cases of child abuse to a child protective service agency. **(PED)**

▶ To prepare for a sigmoidoscopy, the nurse should place the patient in the knee-chest or Sims' position. **(M-S)**

▶ The nurse should suspect sexual abuse in the pediatric patient who presents with unexplained genital trauma or a sexually transmitted disease. **(PED)**

▶ Central venous pressure is the pressure in the right atrium and great veins in the thorax. **(M-S)**

▶ Central venous pressure normally ranges from 2 to 8 mm Hg or 5 to 12 cm H_2O. **(M-S)**

▶ Central venous pressure serves as a guide for assessing right-sided cardiac function. **(M-S)**

▶ Central venous access may be ordered to evaluate circulatory pressure in the right atrium and central veins. **(M-S)**

▶ To administer S.C. heparin (Liquaemin), insert the needle into the skin at a right angle. **(FND)**

▶ For the postoperative patient at risk for deep vein thrombosis, heparin (Liquaemin) or enoxaparin (Lovenox) is usually given. **(M-S)**

▶ Oral anticoagulants, such as warfarin (Coumadin), prevent thrombus formation. **(M-S)**

▶ Anticoagulants can't dissolve a thrombus that has already formed. **(M-S)**

▶ Anticoagulant therapy is contraindicated in patients with severe diabetes, liver or kidney disease, or ulcers. **(M-S)**

▶ To assess a patient for thrombophlebitis, the nurse should compare the measurements of the affected and unaffected limbs every day. **(M-S)**

▶ Before moving the trauma patient, the nurse should ensure that the airway is patent and the cervical spine is immobilized. **(M-S)**

▶ To prepare for a sigmoidoscopy, the nurse should administer an enema 1 hour before the procedure. **(M-S)**

▶ Administering a vasopressor, using an ice water lavage, and inserting an esophageal balloon tamponade are treatments for bleeding esophageal varices. **(M-S)**

▶ After a mastectomy, a symptom of lymphedema is a heavy sensation in the arm. **(M-S)**

▶ It is appropriate for parents to tell their dying child that they will miss the child. **(PED)**

▶ For a school-age child who is dying, the nurse should allow the child to die while being comforted by family members. **(PED)**

▶ For an adolescent who is dying, the nurse should tell the truth about the prognosis but not remove the last "ray of hope." **(PED)**

▶ An adolescent who is dying may be resentful and use denial as a defense mechanism. **(PED)**

▶ When a dying patient asks how much time is left to live, the nurse shouldn't provide an absolute time. **(M-S)**

▶ After the death of a child, the nurse should allow the family to spend time with the body. **(PED)**

► Usually, amniocentesis is done at 12 to 16 weeks' gestation to detect inborn errors of metabolism. **(MAT)**

► Immediate treatment for noncorrosive poisoning of a child over age 1 is 1 tbs (15 ml) of ipecac syrup mixed in 6 to 8 oz (177 to 237 ml) of warm water. **(PED)**

► A sign is an objective indication of a disease that can be perceived by an examiner. **(FND)**

► A symptom is a subjective indication of a disease or condition that is reported by the patient. **(FND)**

► Many alcoholic individuals use alcohol to escape reality. **(PSY)**

► When a fracture is set in a child age 12 and younger, end-to-end apposition of fractured ends isn't essential. **(PED)**

► Celiac disease commonly is diagnosed at age 6 to 24 months. **(PED)**

► Treatment for celiac disease includes consumption of a gluten-free diet for the remainder of the child's life. **(PED)**

► The ultimate nursing goal for the patient with a disability is to assist in reaching the patient's maximum health potential. **(FND)**

► Nitroglycerin tablets are considered expired 5 to 6 months after the bottle has been opened. **(M-S)**

► Physiologic jaundice is common at the beginning of day 2 of life, peaking at one week and disappearing in the second week. **(MAT)**

► Pathologic jaundice is evident in the first 24 hours of life. **(MAT)**

► The puncture (cutdown) site used for cardiac catheterization should be monitored for hematoma formation. **(M-S)**

► When using problem-oriented medical records, the health care team should focus on the patient's problem list. **(FND)**

► Myopia is nearsightedness; hyperopia is farsightedness. **(FND)**

► Nystagmus is the rapid and involuntary horizontal, vertical, or rotating movement of the eyeballs. **(FND)**

► The optic disk is circular, appears yellowish-pink, and has a distinct border. **(FND)**

► When communicating with a child, the nurse should attempt to communicate at eye level. **(PED)**

► The watch-tick test evaluates a patient's ability to hear high frequency sounds. **(M-S)**

▶ The Weber test assesses hearing acuity by way of bone conduction.
(M-S)

▶ The Rinne test evaluates hearing acuity by comparing air and bone conduction.
(M-S)

▶ Signs of pacemaker failure include dizziness, fainting, palpitations, hiccups, and chest pain.
(M-S)

▶ Primary disability results from a disease or disorder.   **(FND)**

▶ When trying to elicit or clarify patient information, the nurse should use open-ended questions.   **(FND)**

▶ The failure rate of a birth control method is expressed as pregnancies per 100 women per year.   **(M-S)**

▶ The anteroposterior diameter is the narrowest diameter of the pelvic inlet.   **(MAT)**

▶ The chorion is the outermost embryonic membrane; it gives rise to the placenta.   **(MAT)**

▶ The amnion is the innermost embryonic membrane.   **(MAT)**

▶ The corpus luteum produces large quantities of progesterone. **(MAT)**

▶ The fetal period of development starts at the eighth week and continues until delivery.   **(MAT)**

▶ Before the patient with an amputation can be fitted for a prosthesis, the residual limb must be shrunk.   **(M-S)**

▶ The patient with rheumatoid arthritis experiences the most severe pain starting in the small joints of the hands, wrists, and feet. **(M-S)**

▶ Autism usually first appears during infancy.   **(PED)**

▶ In an incomplete abortion, the fetus has been expelled but parts of the placenta and amniotic membrane remain in the uterus. **(MAT)**

▶ Normally, a neonate has a head circumference of 13.8″ (35 cm) and a chest circumference of 13″ (33 cm).   **(MAT)**

▶ During the first year, the infant's head and chest circumferences become equal.   **(PED)**

▶ During the first period of reactivity, the newborn is alert, awake, and attentive.   **(MAT)**

▶ The patient with placenta previa and vaginal bleeding should be placed in semi-Fowler's position.   **(MAT)**

▶ Immediately after delivery, establishing a patent airway in the neonate takes highest priority. **(MAT)**

▶ Before getting the patient out of bed for the first time after surgery, the nurse should have the patient dangle his legs over the edge of the bed. **(M-S)**

▶ Greenstick fractures are the most common type of bone fractures in children. **(PED)**

▶ The nurse shouldn't induce vomiting in a patient who has swallowed strychnine, hydrocarbon, or a strong acid or alkali. **(M-S)**

▶ Hydrocarbons can cause severe pneumonia if aspirated. **(M-S)**

▶ Nitroglycerin should cause a slight stinging sensation when placed under the tongue. **(M-S)**

▶ The infant with congenital hip dislocation has a positive Ortolani's sign. **(MAT)**

▶ The patient with cholecystitis may report clay-colored (pale) stools if the common bile duct is obstructed. **(M-S)**

▶ A pacemaker, surgical or orthopedic clips, or shrapnel will interfere with the results of a magnetic resonance imaging scan. **(M-S)**

▶ Benign prostatic hyperplasia typically causes urinary hesitancy and decreases the size and force of the urinary stream. **(M-S)**

▶ Distended neck veins, ankle edema, and unexplained weight gain signal right-sided heart failure. **(M-S)**

▶ In a neonate, tremors or jitteriness may indicate hypoglycemia. **(MAT)**

▶ For neonates with narcotic-induced respiratory depression at birth, naloxone (Narcan), a narcotic antagonist, is the drug of choice. **(MAT)**

▶ Pregnancy-induced hypertension usually resolves shortly after delivery. **(MAT)**

▶ Safety is a primary concern for the person who somnambulates (sleep-walks). **(M-S)**

▶ The optimal schedule for administering an around-the-clock antibiotic is 6 a.m., 12 p.m., 6 p.m., and 12 a.m. **(FND)**

▶ The nurse must follow standard precautions when caring for a patient with hepatitis B. **(FND)**

▶ Obsessive-compulsive patients can't control their behavior and receive no pleasure from it. **(PSY)**

▶ A woman should refrain from getting pregnant for 4 months following an abortion. **(MAT)**

▶ When opening a sterile surgical pack, the nurse should first open the top leaf of the protective towel away from herself. **(FND)**

▶ The nurse should adjust the fingers of sterile gloves only after putting on both gloves. **(FND)**

▶ The nurse should remove sterile gloves before removing a mask because the gloves are more contaminated than the mask. **(FND)**

▶ During a long sterile procedure, a mask that becomes moist should be covered with another sterile mask by someone who isn't in sterile attire. **(FND)**

▶ Activities of daily living include hygiene, elimination, environmental control, comfort measures, nutrition, activity, and mobility. **(FND)**

▶ Following an endoscopy, check the patient for hemoptysis. **(M-S)**

▶ To determine a smoker's pack-year history, the nurse multiplies the number of packs smoked per day by the number of years the person has been smoking. **(FND)**

▶ When caring for the patient with eclampsia who is receiving magnesium sulfate, the nurse should assess for respiratory depression and diminished deep-tendon reflexes. **(MAT)**

▶ The diabetic patient who becomes hypoglycemic should consume an easily digested carbohydrate, such as orange juice or a lump of sugar. **(MAT)**

▶ Amino acids are the end-product of protein digestion. **(M-S)**

▶ The breakdown of glycogen into glucose is called glycogenolysis. **(M-S)**

▶ Insulin is produced by the beta cells of the islets of Langerhans. **(M-S)**

▶ Glucagon is one of the hormones responsible for glycogenolysis. **(M-S)**

▶ Water-soluble vitamins aren't stored by the body. **(M-S)**

▶ Oliguria is the formation and excretion of less than 30 ml of urine an hour, or less than 500 ml during a 24-hour period. **(FND)**

▶ Anuria is the formation and excretion of less than 100 ml of urine in a 24-hour period. **(FND)**

▶ The patient with Parkinson's disease should be instructed to walk with a broad-based gait (with feet apart). **(M-S)**

▶ The patient with myasthenia gravis may have a sleepy, masklike facial expression. **(M-S)**

▶ The nurse should monitor for muscle weakness in the patient with myasthenia gravis who is receiving neostigmine methylsulfate (Prostigmin). **(M-S)**

▶ The patient with myasthenia gravis who experiences diplopia should place an eye patch over one eye and move the head from side to side to enhance the visual field. **(M-S)**

▶ The patient with structural scoliosis should wear a Milwaukee brace 23 hours a day. **(M-S)**

▶ The patient with chronic pancreatitis needs pancreatic enzyme replacement and nutritional supplements. **(M-S)**

▶ The nurse should encourage the patient with diabetes to exercise regularly every day — usually 90 minutes after a meal. **(M-S)**

▶ The patient with a tracheostomy should humidify the air in the home. **(M-S)**

▶ The nurse should instruct the postmastectomy patient to exercise the affected arm to prevent frozen shoulder. **(M-S)**

▶ The woman who has had a unilateral oophorectomy ovulates every other month. **(M-S)**

▶ Cancer spreads by invasion or metastasis. **(M-S)**

▶ The patient with unstable angina experiences pain at rest. **(M-S)**

▶ The patient with a nihilistic delusion denies reality or existence of the self, part of the self, or some external object. **(PSY)**

▶ To measure the amount of liquid medication in a medicine cup, the nurse should hold the medicine cup at eye level and measure at the bottom of the meniscus. **(FND)**

▶ While administering a heparin injection, aspirating for blood return could cause a hematoma. **(M-S)**

▶ If a patient has difficulty swallowing an oral medication, the nurse should advise him to place the medication as far back in his throat as possible. **(FND)**

▶ After administering a vaginal suppository, the nurse should instruct the patient to remain supine for 5 to 10 minutes. **(FND)**

▶ When giving a Z-track injection, the nurse should use the dorsogluteal, ventrogluteal, or vastus lateralis site. **(FND)**

▶ Measles, mumps, and rubella immunization is usually given at age 12 to 15 months. **(PED)**

▶ Atelectasis typically occurs 24 to 48 hours after surgery. **(M-S)**

▶ During the first trimester of pregnancy, the woman should gain 3 to 5 lb (1.4 to 2.3 kg). **(MAT)**

▶ The adverse effects of vincristine (Oncovin) are alopecia, nausea, and vomiting. **(M-S)**

▶ Don't place a pillow under the affected extremity for the patient with hemiplegia as this encourages flexion deformity and impedes circulation. **(M-S)**

▶ When using a cane, the patient should stand erect and carry the cane on the unaffected side. **(M-S)**.

▶ Ensuring patient safety is the nurse's highest priority when caring for the potentially suicidal patient. **(PSY)**

▶ The most common adverse effect of electroconvulsive therapy is postshock amnesia. **(PSY)**

▶ Until regaining consciousness, postoperative patients who received general anesthesia are at risk for aspiration and should be positioned on their sides or have their heads turned to the side if side-lying positions are contraindicated. **(M-S)**

▶ Atropine is given preoperatively to diminish secretions. **(M-S)**

▶ The nurse should advise the patient who has experienced an adverse drug reaction to withhold the next medication dose and call the doctor. **(FND)**

▶ Cervical dilation occurs with true labor and is considered the primary difference between true and false labor. **(MAT)**

▶ The nurse should assess fetal heart tones immediately after the amniotic membranes rupture. **(MAT)**

▶ The patient receiving epidural anesthesia during labor should be placed on her side with her head slightly raised. **(MAT)**

▶ Skin color changes in dark-skinned persons can best be seen in areas of less pigmentation, such as lips, mucous membranes, ear lobes, palms, and soles. **(M-S)**

▶ Raisins are a good snack for the child with iron deficiency anemia; eating vegetables every day is also recommended. **(PED)**

▶ When working with the schizophrenic patient, the nurse must gain the patient's trust. **(PSY)**

▶ Before removing a urinary catheter that has been in place for a prolonged period, the nurse should clamp the catheter several times each day. **(M-S)**

▶ The neonate who weighs 7 lb (3.2 kg) at birth should weigh 14 lb (6.4 kg) by age 6 months and 21 lb (9.5 kg) by age 12 months. **(MAT)**

▶ A gluten-free diet allows rice but excludes such foods as oats, wheat, and barley. **(M-S)**

▶ Accidents are the leading cause of death in children ages 1 to 4. **(PED)**

▶ The child playing alone with toys that differ from those used by nearby children is engaging in solitary play. **(PED)**

▶ Parallel play typically is seen in toddlers who play independently but alongside other children. **(PED)**

▶ Tay-Sachs disease occurs mainly in Ashkenazi (eastern European) Jews and is manifested by cherry-red spots on the macula. **(M-S)**

▶ Fraternal (dizygotic) twins derive from the fertilization of two separate ova. **(MAT)**

▶ Identical (monozygotic) twins derive from the fertilization of one ovum. **(MAT)**

▶ Monozygotic twins have an identical genetic makeup. **(MAT)**

▶ Dizygotic twins have separate and distinct placentas and membranes. **(MAT)**

▶ A fetal teratogen is any agent or substance capable of causing an adverse effect in the developing fetus. **(MAT)**

▶ An infant's breathing is primarily abdominal. **(MAT)**

▶ A rectal thermometer typically has a blunt, rounded bulb; an oral thermometer has a slender, elongated tip. **(FND)**

▶ Marbling and speckling of the iris (called Brushfield's spots) are seen in children with Down syndrome.   **(PED)**

▶ The newborn female may have pseudomenstruation.   **(MAT)**

▶ The normal umbilical cord consists of two arteries and one vein.   **(MAT)**

▶ Vitamin K is administered to neonates shortly after birth to prevent hemorrhage.   **(MAT)**

▶ A fractured clavicle (collarbone) is a common birth injury in large-for-gestational-age neonates.   **(MAT)**

▶ The therapeutic range of digoxin is 0.5 to 2 mg/ml.   **(M-S)**

▶ If the pregnant patient becomes dizzy on the examination table, the nurse should place the patient on her left side.   **(MAT)**

▶ Immediately after delivery, the neonate should be suctioned to ensure an adequate airway and normal breathing.   **(MAT)**

▶ The nurse should keep calcium gluconate 10% at the bedside of the patient receiving magnesium sulfate for administration if signs of respiratory depression develop.   **(M-S)**

▶ Estriol determination is used to assess placental function and fetal well-being.   **(MAT)**

▶ If the fetus has a prolapsed umbilical cord, the nurse should place the mother in Trendelenburg's or the knee-chest position with her hips elevated.   **(MAT)**

▶ A variation from the normal fetal heart rate pattern may indicate fetal distress.   **(MAT)**

▶ Pelvic thrombophlebitis most commonly occurs about 2 weeks after delivery.   **(M-S)**

▶ The most common cause of postpartum hemorrhage is uterine atony.   **(MAT)**

▶ Signs of tracheoesophageal fistula in the neonate include excessive nasal secretions, drooling, and violent choking during feeding.   **(MAT)**

▶ Respiratory distress syndrome is common in premature neonates.   **(MAT)**

▶ To reduce the risk of aspiration, the nurse should feed the infant with a cleft lip or palate in an upright position.   **(MAT)**

▶ If water accumulates in the tubing of an oxygen delivery system line, the nurse should disconnect the tubing and empty the water. **(M-S)**

▶ Before administering morphine sulfate, the nurse should check the patient's respiratory rate; if it is less than 12 breaths/minute, the nurse should withhold the drug and call the doctor. **(M-S)**

▶ A temporary drainage appliance is placed on a new ileostomy as soon as surgery ends. **(M-S)**

▶ Laboratory values elevated following a myocardial infarction include creatine kinase, CK-MB, and lactate dehydrogenase-1. **(M-S)**

▶ The child experiencing night terrors awakens screaming and can't recall what caused the frightening episode. **(PED)**

▶ Narcolepsy is characterized by an uncontrollable desire to sleep. **(M-S)**

▶ Bruxism is unconscious grinding or clenching of the teeth, especially during sleep. **(M-S)**

▶ Chronic pain is limited, intermittent, or persistent pain of more than 6 months' duration. **(FND)**

▶ Acute pain is transient pain of sudden onset, varying intensity, and less than 6 months' duration. **(FND)**

▶ Signs and symptoms of acute myelogenous leukemia include increased susceptibility to infection, weakness, fatigue, bleeding, and enlarged lymph nodes. **(M-S)**

▶ In acute myelogenous leukemia, bleeding results from decreased platelet production. **(M-S)**

▶ The nurse should avoid palpating the abdomen of the child with Wilms' tumor because palpation could cause metastasis. **(PED)**

▶ The patient taking anticoagulants as an outpatient should be instructed to call the doctor if he passes black, tarry stools. **(M-S)**

▶ The nurse should reassure parents that breast engorgement is normal in neonates. **(MAT)**

▶ The first deciduous teeth to erupt in an infant are the lower central incisors. **(PED)**

▶ The two major stages of sleep are non–rapid-eye-movement and rapid-eye-movement sleep. **(M-S)**

▶ The neonate's posterior fontanel may not be visible at delivery because of molding; it usually closes by age 2 to 3 months.   **(MAT)**

▶ The mature ovum and sperm each contain 23 chromosomes. **(MAT)**

▶ Sperm retain their fertilizing capability for at least 48 hours after sexual intercourse.   **(MAT)**

▶ The joint action of luteinizing hormone and follicle-stimulating hormone cause the ovarian follicle to mature.   **(MAT)**

▶ Women should perform breast self-examination at least every month, approximately 1 week after menses.   **(M-S)**

▶ Men should check their testicles for masses at least every month, preferably during a warm shower or bath.   **(M-S)**

▶ Early signs of croup can be managed at home by placing the child in a closed bathroom and running hot water in the shower or bathtub.   **(PED)**

▶ A low-calcium diet is prescribed for patients at increased risk for renal calculi (such as immobilized patients).   **(M-S)**

▶ One gram of protein contains 4 calories.   **(FND)**

▶ Vitamin K deficiency may affect blood coagulation.   **(M-S)**

▶ The post-prostatectomy patient receiving estrogen may experience breast enlargement (gynecomastia).   **(M-S)**

▶ If the patient on a respirator becomes restless, he may need suctioning.   **(M-S)**

▶ The body stores glucose as glycogen.   **(M-S)**

▶ Broccoli, cabbage, and collard greens are high in calcium.   **(M-S)**

▶ During the fight or flight reaction, release of glucagon and epinephrine is responsible for glycogen conversion to glucose.   **(PSY)**

▶ To prevent rickets, a person must consume adequate amounts of calcium and vitamin D.   **(M-S)**

▶ In the neonate, respiratory distress causes nasal flaring, see-saw retractions, and expiratory grunting.   **(MAT)**

▶ For the patient with chronic obstructive pulmonary disease, high oxygen levels inhibit the respiratory drive.   **(M-S)**

▶ The patient who breathes out while the mechanical ventilator is on the inspiratory cycle is said to be "fighting" the ventilator.   **(M-S)**

▶ The nurse should monitor the partial thromboplastin time of the patient receiving heparin. **(M-S)**

▶ During the orientation phase of the therapeutic relationship, patients commonly display testing and resistive behavior. **(FND)**

▶ Postmenopausal bleeding is a common sign of uterine cancer. **(M-S)**

▶ The most common sign of laryngeal cancer is hoarseness or a change in the voice. **(M-S)**

▶ Pain radiating to the left shoulder from the splenic region suggests splenic rupture. **(M-S)**

▶ To prevent plantar flexion in the bedridden patient, the nurse should use a footboard or have the patient wear high-top athletic shoes. **(M-S)**

▶ Nocturnal enuresis (involuntary urination during sleep) typically occurs during stage II of non–rapid-eye-movement sleep. **(M-S)**

▶ The nurse should instruct the patient with gout to avoid organ meats such as liver because of their high purine content. **(M-S)**

▶ A trochanter roll should extend from the crest of the ilium to the mid-thigh. **(M-S)**

▶ To determine if the patient has a pulse deficit, one nurse should measure the apical pulse while a second nurse measures the radial pulse at the same time, using the same watch. **(FND)**

▶ The patient with hypothyroidism can't tolerate cold. **(M-S)**

▶ The patient with hyperthyroidism can't tolerate heat. **(M-S)**

▶ The nurse should make sure the patient is dried thoroughly after a bath. **(FND)**

▶ When a toddler is hospitalized, the nurse should ask the parents about the child's sleep rituals. **(PED)**

▶ To help assess the patient's judgment, the nurse should ask such questions as, "If you found a stamped, addressed envelope, what would you do with it?". **(FND)**

▶ After a bone marrow aspiration, the nurse should apply pressure to the puncture site for 5 to 10 minutes to ensure hemostasis. **(M-S)**

▶ In an immunosuppressed patient, the patient's own microorganisms are the most common cause of infection. **(M-S)**

▶ A T tube is inserted into the common bile duct after a cholecystectomy to allow drainage of bile. **(M-S)**

▶ Sharp pain in the right upper abdominal quadrant that radiates to the back or right shoulder is a common sign of cholecystitis. **(M-S)**

▶ Before a cholangiogram, the nurse should assess the patient for allergies, especially to iodine or shellfish. **(M-S)**

▶ An oral cholangiogram is used only if ultrasound is unavailable or yields inconclusive results. **(M-S)**

▶ The patient scheduled for a cholecystogram should take oral dye tablets 2 to 3 hours after the evening meal on the night before the test, or 10 to 12 hours before the test. **(M-S)**

▶ During I.V. cholangiography, I.V. radioactive isotopes are injected. **(M-S)**

▶ Adverse reactions to contrast media range from nausea and vomiting to hives and anaphylactic shock. **(M-S)**

▶ If Rocky Mountain spotted fever is suspected, the nurse should ask if the patient has been in the woods lately or been bitten by a tick. **(M-S)**

▶ Having the patient say "ahhh" when obtaining a throat culture relaxes the throat muscles and diminishes the gag reflex. **(FND)**

▶ The nurse should obtain a specimen for a wound culture from the wound drainage area. **(M-S)**

▶ One tablespoon of a stool is usually sufficient for laboratory analysis. **(FND)**

▶ Normal vaginal or urethral discharge is clear or white, contains no pus or blood, and is minimal. **(M-S)**

▶ The nurse shouldn't withhold oral intake before an EEG because the resulting hypoglycemia may alter test results. **(M-S)**

▶ Before an EEG, the patient's hair and scalp should be shampooed. **(M-S)**

▶ The patient with pernicious anemia commonly experiences hypochlorhydria or achlorhydria. **(M-S)**

▶ Persistent obstruction of the portal venous circulation almost always leads to esophageal varices. **(M-S)**

▶ After an upper GI endoscopy, the patient should receive nothing by mouth until a normal gag reflex returns. **(M-S)**

▶ The patient who has undergone an upper GI endoscopy may have slightly bloody sputum if a tissue biopsy sample was obtained from an area high in the esophagus. **(M-S)**

▶ On the morning before an upper GI X-ray, the nurse should instruct the patient not to smoke or chew gum because these actions stimulate gastric motility. **(M-S)**

▶ After an upper GI X-ray, the nurse should instruct the patient to increase fluid intake and eat a high-fiber diet to promote barium passage. **(M-S)**

▶ Glucose breaks down into carbon dioxide and water. **(M-S)**

▶ The nurse should instruct the diabetic patient to check his blood glucose level before each meal and at bedtime. **(M-S)**

▶ When performing a fingerstick blood glucose test, the nurse should blot away the first blood drop because it may be diluted by body fluids. **(M-S)**

▶ Before a contrast medium injection, the nurse should tell the patient to expect a transient burning sensation and a metallic taste in his mouth. **(M-S)**

▶ Normal cerebrospinal fluid is clear and colorless. **(M-S)**

▶ The patient should lie flat in bed for at least 8 hours after a lumbar puncture. **(M-S)**

▶ If the patient's cerebrospinal fluid pressure rises after a lumbar puncture, the nurse should take vital signs and perform a neurologic assessment every 15 minutes for the first 4 hours, then every hour for the next 2 hours. **(M-S)**

▶ Postmenopausal women should perform breast self-examination each month, on the same day of the month. **(M-S)**

▶ Following cataract removal, the patient should avoid bending over, coughing, or engaging in any activity that increases intraocular pressure. **(M-S)**

▶ The patient who has had a myelogram followed by removal of a non-water-soluble agent must return to the room on a stretcher and must lie flat. **(M-S)**

▶ The nurse should clean a child's ear with a soft cloth before examining it. **(PED)**

▶ When examining the ear of an adult, the nurse should pull the auricle up and back to straighten the ear canal. **(M-S)**

▶ After eardrop instillation, the patient should lie on his side for 5 to 10 minutes. **(M-S)**

▶ The nurse should instill eyedrops into the conjunctiva to prevent damage to the cornea and apply ointment on the edge of the conjunctival sac. **(M-S)**

▶ Cancer can occur anywhere in the colon but is most commonly found in the rectum and sigmoid colon. **(M-S)**

▶ A change in bowel habits is the most common presenting sign of colon cancer. **(M-S)**

▶ The patient with ulcerative colitis should eat a low-residue, high-protein diet. **(M-S)**

▶ Placing one hand on the throat is the universal sign of choking. **(M-S)**

▶ The patient's identification bracelet should stay in place until he leaves the hospital grounds. **(FND)**

▶ The most reliable way to identify the patient is to check the identification bracelet. **(FND)**

▶ The nurse should begin discharge planning when the patient is admitted. **(FND)**

▶ During the patient's hospital orientation, the staff should demonstrate proper use of the call bell system. **(FND)**

▶ Clonus is rapidly alternating involuntary muscle contraction and relaxation. **(M-S)**

▶ Before ambulating the patient who needs ambulatory assistive aids, the nurse should first explain the procedure and then assemble the necessary equipment. **(M-S)**

▶ Dangling the patient's legs before getting him out of bed helps to prevent pooling of blood and orthostatic hypotension. **(M-S)**

▶ The postoperative patient should receive pain medication 30 minutes before ambulating. **(M-S)**

▶ If the patient has weakness on one side of the body, the nurse should stand on the weak side to provide support during rising and ambulation. **(M-S)**

▶ The nurse should place the patient's bed in the lowest position after giving a bed bath and performing other care activities. **(M-S)**

▶ The patient with hemiplegia should have his position changed at least every 2 hours and should be placed mainly on the unaffected side with only brief periods on the affected side. **(M-S)**

▶ Water for a bed bath should be heated to 110° to 115° F (43.3° to 46° C). **(FND)**

▶ A fiberglass cast dries immediately after application. **(M-S)**

▶ A therapeutic bath contains an additive, such as oatmeal, cornstarch, sodium bicarbonate, oil, or a medication. **(FND)**

▶ To avoid transmitting microorganisms, the nurse should avoid direct contact between the nurse's uniform and the patient's bed linens. **(FND)**

▶ Rolling the patient toward the nurse when moving the bedridden patient in bed reduces strain and exertion. **(M-S)**

▶ Until a plaster cast is completely dry, the nurse should handle it with the palms of her hands. **(M-S)**

▶ An extremity with a plaster cast should be turned every 2 hours to promote even drying. **(M-S)**

▶ Cystitis, an inflammation of the urinary bladder, most commonly results from an infection that ascends from the urethra. **(M-S)**

▶ Candidiasis is a fungal infection caused by *Candida albicans*. **(M-S)**

▶ The nurse should tape the indwelling urinary catheter of a female patient to the patient's leg. **(M-S)**

▶ When inserting a urinary catheter in a male patient, the nurse should raise the penis to an angle of 60 to 90 degrees. **(M-S)**

▶ The practical nurse should complete only the original copy of an incident report and then submit the report to a registered nurse. **(FND)**

▶ The pregnant patient who has poor balance should take showers instead of baths. **(MAT)**

▶ Respiratory depression is a common adverse effect of morphine. **(M-S)**

▶ Macronutrients are essential nutrients that supply energy and build tissue; they include carbohydrates, fats, and proteins. **(M-S)**

▶ Green, leafy vegetables are good sources of magnesium. **(M-S)**

▶ Metabolism is the chemical changes within the body that make energy available. **(M-S)**

▶ If the patient is using a hand-held inhaler, the nurse should instruct him to wait 30 to 60 seconds after the first puff before taking a second puff. **(M-S)**

▶ To drain the apical sections of the upper lung lobes using postural drainage, the nurse should have the patient sit in high Fowler's position. **(M-S)**

▶ On percussion, areas containing air or gas produce tympany, a drumlike sound. **(FND)**

▶ Black or tarry stools are associated with upper GI bleeding or a diet high in red meat or dark, green vegetables. **(M-S)**

▶ Before collecting a stool specimen, the nurse should instruct the patient to urinate. **(M-S)**

▶ For best results, the patient should retain an oil-retention enema for at least 30 minutes. **(M-S)**

▶ When obtaining a urine sample from an indwelling urinary catheter, the nurse should clamp the tubing and allow the urine to collect and then insert a 21G to 25G 1″ needle through an injection port. **(M-S)**

▶ The normal ratio of carbonic acids to bicarbonate ions is 1:20. **(M-S)**

▶ To measure the amount of urine in a diaper, the nurse should subtract the weight of a dry diaper from the weight of the wet diaper and convert the number of grams to milliliters (1 gram to 1 milliliter). **(PED)**

▶ The anion gap is the difference between the concentrations of serum anions and cations determined by subtracting the sum of chloride and bicarbonate anions from sodium cations. **(M-S)**

▶ Microdrip I.V. tubing delivers 60 drops/ml. **(M-S)**

▶ Macrodrip I.V. tubing delivers 10, 15, 20, or 30 drops/ml, depending on the manufacturer. **(M-S)**

▶ Sodium is the major cation in extracellular fluid. **(M-S)**

▶ To prevent vomiting, postural drainage should be performed 1 to 2 hours after the patient eats a meal. **(M-S)**

▶ Tidal volume is the amount of air inspired and expired in a normal respiration. **(M-S)**

▶ Surfactant is a mixture of lipoproteins in the lungs that reduces the surface tension of pulmonary fluids. **(M-S)**

▶ Hemoglobin is an oxygen-carrying pigment in red blood cells. **(M-S)**

▶ Kussmaul respirations are associated with metabolic acidosis. **(M-S)**

▶ Abnormal breath sounds are called adventitious. **(M-S)**

▶ An incentive spirometer is sometimes called a sustained maximal inspiration device. **(M-S)**

▶ When teaching pursed-lip breathing, the nurse should instruct the patient to inhale through the nose and then exhale slowly and evenly against pursed lips while tightening the abdominal muscles. **(M-S)**

▶ Infants have a higher proportion of body fluids than other age-groups. **(PED)**

▶ Body fat contains a small amount of water, whereas lean tissue is rich in water. **(M-S)**

▶ Women have proportionally more body fat, and therefore less body fluid, than men. **(M-S)**

▶ Sebum is the fatty secretion of a sebaceous gland. **(M-S)**

▶ Diffusion is the movement of a solute from an area of higher concentration to an area of lower concentration. **(M-S)**

▶ Osmosis is the movement of water across a semipermeable membrane from a less concentrated solution to a more concentrated one. **(M-S)**

▶ Active transport is the movement of a solute across a concentration gradient; it requires energy. **(M-S)**

▶ Hydrostatic pressure is the pressure exerted by a liquid against the walls of a container within a closed system. **(M-S)**

▶ Thoracic breathing is costal, whereas abdominal breathing is diaphragmatic. **(M-S)**

▶ Respiratory depth is described as normal, deep, or shallow. **(FND)**

▶ A normal inspiration lasts 1 to 1½ seconds; a normal expiration lasts 2 to 3 seconds. **(FND)**

▶ In a pureed diet, food is blended to a semisolid consistency. **(M-S)**

▶ When serving meals to a blind patient, the nurse should think of the plate as a clock and place foods at specific times. **(FND)**

▶ A clear liquid diet provides fluid and electrolytes but lacks adequate fats, proteins, vitamins, calories, and minerals. **(M-S)**

▶ Before feeding the patient, the nurse should ask if he prefers to eat foods in any particular order. **(FND)**

▶ The typical large-bore nasogastric tube is a #12 to #14 French tube. **(FND)**

▶ The patient at risk for aspiration should receive an intestinal tube rather than a gastric tube. **(M-S)**

▶ The nurse should check nasogastric tube placement every 4 to 6 hours. **(M-S)**

▶ A large-bore nasogastric (NG) tube is more likely than a small-bore NG tube to cause coughing or choking when it enters the respiratory tract. **(M-S)**

▶ Total body water accounts for approximately 75% of the neonate's weight. **(FND)**

▶ Dextrose 5% in water, lactated Ringer's solution, and normal saline solution are examples of isotonic solutions. **(FND)**

▶ Half-normal saline solution is an example of a hypotonic solution. **(FND)**

▶ An example of a hypertonic solution is 50% glucose. **(FND)**

▶ Fluid loss is termed insensible when it isn't noticeable. Such loss includes fluid lost from the skin through evaporation and fluid lost from the lungs as moisture exhaled through the breath. **(FND)**

▶ Chyme is a semifluid material produced by food digestion in the stomach. **(FND)**

▶ The most common cause of pulmonary edema is left-sided heart failure. **(M-S)**

▶ Diuretic use is the leading cause of potassium deficit. **(M-S)**

▶ Potassium is the major cation in intracellular fluid. **(M-S)**

▶ Instruct the patient with tuberculosis to cover his mouth with a tissue when coughing and to dispose of tissues as biological waste. **(M-S)**

▶ Signs of tension pneumothorax include rapid, shallow respirations, chest pain, and cyanosis. **(M-S)**

▶ A lung is normally fully expanded 1- to 3-days postoperative of chest drainage. **(M-S)**

▶ The elderly patient who becomes confused as night approaches is experiencing sundowner syndrome. **(M-S)**

▶ A Denis Browne splint is used for the child with clubfoot. **(PED)**

▶ Keep two rubber-tipped clamps available for immediate use if chest-tube clamping is required. **(M-S)**

▶ The sinoatrial node is the heart's natural pacemaker. **(M-S)**

▶ The T wave represents repolarization of the ventricles. **(M-S)**

▶ During wound care, the nurse should wear clean gloves when removing the top dressing to avoid exposure to bacteria. **(M-S)**

▶ Functional nursing focuses on tasks and procedures. **(FND)**

▶ An autocratic leader assumes complete control over decisions involving the group. **(FND)**

▶ In the dark-skinned patient, the nurse should check for jaundice by inspecting the hard palate. **(M-S)**

▶ Fat digestion occurs mainly in the small intestine. **(M-S)**

▶ Carbohydrate digestion starts in the mouth. **(M-S)**

▶ Surgical asepsis is the practice of keeping an area or objects free of microorganisms and spores. **(FND)**

▶ Metamucil should be mixed in water before swallowing. **(M-S)**

▶ Check skin turgor above the umbilicus on an infant. **(PED)**

▶ Before applying antiembolism stockings, the nurse should have the patient lie down for 20 minutes with his feet elevated. **(M-S)**

▶ Osteoporosis is a demineralization process in which bones become less dense. **(M-S)**

▶ Having the patient ambulate is the best way to prevent osteoporosis. **(M-S)**

▶ To assess the patient for dehydration, the nurse should check skin turgor. **(M-S)**

▶ Chest tubes should be removed if fluid drainage is less than 50 to 70 ml (1¾ to 2½ oz) daily. **(M-S)**

▶ Sleep apnea (cessation of breathing during sleep) is commonly associated with snoring. **(M-S)**

▶ After a diagnostic study in which the femoral site is used, the patient must lie flat for 8 hours. **(M-S)**

▶ When caring for the patient who has just had a cardiac catheterization, the nurse immediately must report a rapid or irregular pulse. **(M-S)**

▶ The immobilized patient should eat a diet high in protein, calories, and bulk, with liberal amounts of fluid. **(M-S)**

▶ The best method of determining lung reexpansion is chest X-ray; other methods include auscultation and percussion. **(M-S)**

▶ A high alpha-fetoprotein level after the 14th week of gestation is associated with spinal cord defects. **(MAT)**

▶ Autonomy implies freedom, self-control, and the ability to make independent decisions. **(FND)**

▶ Third spacing refers to the shifting of body fluids into a space that normally doesn't contain fluid. **(M-S)**

▶ The characteristic pattern of Guillain-Barré syndrome is ascending weakness starting in the lower extremities and spreading upward to trunk, upper extremities, and face. **(M-S)**

▶ False imprisonment is the unjustifiable retention or prevention of the patient's movement without proper consent or authority. **(FND)**

▶ Euthanasia is the deliberate termination of a person's life. **(FND)**

▶ A living will specifies the medical care the person would consent to or refuse if he lacked the capacity to consent to or refuse treatment. **(FND)**

▶ The neonate should pass meconium in 24 to 48 hours after birth. **(MAT)**

▶ Chvostek's sign is associated with hypocalcemia and hypoparathyroidism. **(M-S)**

▶ The patient receiving lithium carbonate should maintain an adequate salt and fluid intake. **(PSY)**

▶ The patient with glaucoma may complain of seeing a halo around lights or visual images. **(M-S)**

▶ Yellowing of vision is a symptom of digoxin toxicity. **(M-S)**

▶ Hemianopsia is the loss of one side of the visual field. **(M-S)**

▶ To help the patient compensate for loss of peripheral vision, the nurse should have him turn his head slowly to increase the visual field. **(M-S)**

▶ During an enema, the patient may suffer cramps if water flows into the colon too rapidly. **(M-S)**

▶ The patient with carbon monoxide poisoning may have cherry-red or pale, cyanotic skin. **(M-S)**

▶ Credé's maneuver is used to help empty the bladder of the patient with urinary retention. **(M-S)**

▶ The patient with a history of basal cell carcinoma should avoid prolonged exposure to the sun. **(M-S)**

▶ During a bath, the nurse should prevent the patient from becoming chilled. **(FND)**

▶ The neonate's transitional stools are loose and green to yellow. **(MAT)**

▶ By the fourth day after birth, the breast-fed neonate usually passes 3 to 4 light yellow stools daily. **(MAT)**

▶ During phototherapy, the neonate's stools are bright green from increased bilirubin excretion. **(MAT)**

▶ The patient with a C5 spinal injury is able to lift his shoulder and elbow to a limited degree and has no sensation below the clavicle. **(M-S)**

▶ When cleaning a wound, the nurse should wipe in only one direction, using a new gauze pad each time. **(M-S)**

▶ Digoxin causes a slower, stronger heartbeat and allows the heart to rest between beats. **(M-S)**

▶ "Tet spells" are common in children with tetralogy of Fallot. **(PED)**

▶ Neonates usually undergo phenylketonuria testing about 72 hours after birth, after consuming protein. **(MAT)**

▶ Stomach acid turns litmus paper pink or red. **(M-S)**

▶ The nurse should use nitrazine paper to determine if fluid leakage from a pregnant woman is amniotic. **(MAT)**

▶ The Tensilon (edrophonium) test is used to diagnose myasthenia gravis. **(M-S)**

▶ In the child with strabismus, the nondiverging eye should be patched. **(PED)**

▶ Colchicine is the drug of choice for treating acute gout. **(M-S)**

▶ To perform quadriceps sitting exercises, the patient tries to push the popliteal area into the bed while raising the heel. **(M-S)**

▶ Frequent swallowing after a tonsillectomy indicates bleeding of the operative site. **(M-S)**

▶ A xenograft is a skin graft made of tissue from another species. **(M-S)**

▶ A sputum smear and culture provide a definitive diagnosis of tuberculosis. **(M-S)**

▶ The person who tests positive for human immunodeficiency virus shouldn't keep a cat because of the risk of toxoplasmosis transmission. **(M-S)**

▶ Fat embolism usually occurs about 48 hours after a fracture. **(M-S)**

▶ Complete protein foods, such as meat, dairy, fish, poultry, and eggs, contain adequate amounts of the nine essential amino acids. **(M-S)**

▶ In cheilosis, associated with riboflavin deficiency, cracks appear at the corners of the mouth. **(M-S)**

▶ A bland diet may include such foods as milk, cream, cereals, soup, rice, lean meats, fish, custards, and plain cake. **(M-S)**

▶ Rotating tourniquets may be used in the patient with pulmonary edema or severe heart failure. **(M-S)**

▶ Neonates of mothers who smoke are more likely to be small for gestational age than those of nonsmoking mothers. **(MAT)**

▶ When caring for the patient with chest tubes attached to suction, the nurse should keep a clamp at the bedside in case of emergency. **(M-S)**

▶ Viability refers to the ability of a fetus to live outside the womb. **(MAT)**

▶ A high-risk pregnancy is one in which certain conditions, such as age or systemic disease, place the fetus or mother at increased risk for harm or adverse outcome. **(MAT)**

▶ Quickening is a presumptive sign of pregnancy. **(MAT)**

▶ Braxton Hicks contractions are a probable sign of pregnancy. **(MAT)**

▶ Signs of preeclampsia include edema, proteinuria, and increased blood pressure. **(MAT)**

▶ Magnesium sulfate is the drug of choice for patients with pregnancy-induced hypertension. **(MAT)**

▶ A bounding pulse indicates fluid volume excess. **(M-S)**

▶ If the patient has frostbite, the nurse should gradually rewarm the affected part rather than massage the frozen extremities, fingers, or toes. **(M-S)**

▶ The nurse should teach the patient with a colostomy to gently lift the stoma appliance away from the stoma, permitting gas to escape. **(M-S)**

▶ Cretinism is a congenital form of hypothyroidism. **(M-S)**

▶ Respirations are maintained with a phrenic pacemaker in the patient with a C1 or C2 injury. **(M-S)**

▶ Gynecomastia is overdeveloped breast tissue in a male. **(M-S)**

▶ Muscle weakness and cardiac arrhythmia are common complaints in patients with hypokalemia or hyperkalemia. **(M-S)**

▶ A bruit or a rushing sound heard with a stethoscope over the patient's thyroid gland indicates a hypermetabolic state. **(FND)**

▶ Pain is usually a late symptom of colon cancer. **(M-S)**

▶ To conserve energy in the patient who is in a weakened state, the nurse may need to alternate care procedures with rest periods. **(M-S)**

▶ Blood samples drawn before breakfast are usually more chemically uniform than those drawn later in the day. **(M-S)**

▶ The nurse should use a 21G to 23G needle to withdraw blood. **(FND)**

▶ When cleaning a puncture site before a needle aspiration, the nurse should clean from the center outward, using a circular motion. **(FND)**

▶ Slides of material obtained from a bone marrow aspiration must be sent uncontaminated to the laboratory immediately. **(FND)**

▶ After a bone marrow aspiration, the nurse should apply direct pressure to the aspiration site for 5 to 10 minutes. **(M-S)**

▶ The drugs commonly used in the treatment of myasthenia gravis are anticholinesterase medications such as pyridostigmine (Mestinon). **(M-S)**

▶ Before bronchoscopy, the nurse should check the patient for dentures and remove them. **(M-S)**

▶ After bronchoscopy, the nurse should withhold foods and fluids until the patient's gag reflex returns. **(M-S)**

▶ Pain, difficulty swallowing, and an elevated temperature may indicate perforation in the patient who has undergone esophageal endoscopy. **(M-S)**

▶ Obesity is associated with increased insulin resistance. **(M-S)**

▶ Oral antidiabetic agents stimulate insulin production. **(M-S)**

▶ Insulin is destroyed by gastric juices when taken by mouth. **(M-S)**

▶ Exercise lowers the blood glucose level by increasing insulin uptake by muscles and improving insulin utilization. **(M-S)**

▶ Constant motor activity in the patient taking antipsychotic medications is a classic sign of akathisia. **(PSY)**

▶ A neologism is a meaningless word or term coined by a person with a psychosis. **(PSY)**

▶ To administer gavage feedings to an infant, the nurse should use a gravity drip. **(PED)**

▶ An oral airway should be kept at the bedside of the patient on seizure precautions. **(M-S)**

▶ Enterobiasis (also called pinworms) is most commonly diagnosed from a complaint of anal itching. **(M-S)**

▶ A low-fat diet is appropriate for the patient with cholecystitis. **(M-S)**

▶ A decreased vitamin K level causes a prolonged prothrombin time. **(M-S)**

▶ Hydroxyzine pamoate (Vistaril) is given preoperatively to reduce the patient's narcotic requirements and to reduce anxiety. **(M-S)**

▶ Advise the patient taking metronidazole (Flagyl) that he may experience a metallic taste in his mouth and dark red-brown urine. **(M-S)**

▶ Correcting electrolyte imbalances is the priority nursing goal for the patient with anorexia nervosa. **(PSY)**

▶ To prevent self-induced vomiting, the nurse should monitor the patient with anorexia nervosa for 45 to 90 minutes after meals. **(PSY)**

▶ A dry delivery occurs when the fetus isn't delivered within 24 hours after rupture of the amniotic membranes. **(MAT)**

▶ If the doctor orders 5 lb (2.3 kg) of traction weight for the child in Bryant's traction, the nurse should place 2½-lb weights on each leg. **(PED)**

▶ For the child in Bryant's traction, a vest jacket or an abdominal restraint is used instead of elbow restraints. **(PED)**

▶ A mobile provides visual stimulation only and should be removed from the infant's bed when he reaches age 4 months. **(PED)**

▶ For the 5-year-old child confined to bed, effective diversional activities include playing with clay and drawing. **(PED)**

▶ The patient receiving disulfiram (Antabuse) should avoid alcohol and alcohol-containing products. **(M-S)**

▶ Disulfiram serves as aversion therapy for patients desiring to abstain from alcohol. **(PSY)**

▶ The nurse should administer lithium carbonate with meals to minimize GI upset. **(PSY)**

▶ Methylene blue (Urolene Blue) can turn the urine (and sometimes the stool) blue-green. **(M-S)**

▶ If the patient's hair is matted with blood, clean it with hydrogen peroxide to dissolve the blood and then rinse it with saline solution. **(M-S)**

▶ Before and after administering a narcotic, the nurse must assess the patient for respiratory depression. **(M-S)**

▶ The nurse should irrigate the patient's eye from the inner canthus to the outer canthus. **(M-S)**

▶ Before applying an eye ointment, the nurse should express a small amount of ointment onto a sterile gauze pad. **(M-S)**

▶ A bed cradle is used to keep bed sheets and blankets off the patient's feet. **(M-S)**

▶ The three domains of learning are psychomotor, cognitive, and affective. **(FND)**

▶ The neonatal period encompasses the first 28 days after birth. **(PED)**

▶ Fixation refers to arrested development of the personality at a particular stage because of anxiety. **(PSY)**

▶ At birth, the neonate's hearing is indistinct because of fluid retention in the middle ear. **(MAT)**

▶ Meconium is the first fecal material passed by the neonate. **(MAT)**

▶ Normal urine output for a neonate is 15 to 60 ml (½ to 2 oz) per day. **(MAT)**

▶ Children under age 6 who have a history of pica are at risk for lead poisoning. **(PED)**

▶ The four types of play are onlooker play, solitary play, parallel play, and associative play. **(PED)**

▶ The ability to identify an object by touch is called stereognosis. **(FND)**

▶ Regression means a return to an earlier stage of development. **(PED)**

▶ Ovulation typically occurs 1 to 2 years after menarche. **(M-S)**

▶ To prevent anemia, females ages 10 to 55 should consume 18 mg of iron daily. **(M-S)**

▶ Menopause is the cessation of menses. **(M-S)**

▶ Climacteric is the cessation of reproductive functioning in women (menopause) and decreasing testicular action in men. **(M-S)**

▶ Hot flashes may take the form of sweating, heat sensation in the chest, sleep disturbance, or chills. **(M-S)**

▶ Lentigo senilis, sometimes called "age spots" or "liver spots," result from melanocyte clustering. **(M-S)**

▶ According to the continuity theory, individuals maintain their values, morals, behavior, and habits as they age. **(FND)**

▶ For optimal effectiveness, the nurse should administer antacids 1 hour after meals. **(M-S)**

▶ Bone marrow suppression is a life-threatening risk associated with phenytoin (Dilantin) therapy. **(M-S)**

▶ The patient who takes insulin should avoid alcohol and aspirin unless the doctor approves. **(M-S)**

▶ The nurse should warn the patient on antipsychotic drug therapy to avoid activities that require alertness or good psychomotor control and to apply sunscreen before engaging in outdoor daylight activities that expose him to the sun. **(PSY)**

▶ Withdrawal symptoms may occur in the patient who abruptly stops taking barbiturates after long-term use. **(M-S)**

▶ To relieve dry mouth, the nurse should provide sugarless hard candy, a mouth rinse, ice chips, or glycerine swabs (unless contraindicated). **(M-S)**

▶ The patient with a serum potassium level below 3 mEq/L needs potassium replacement therapy. **(M-S)**

▶ Thyroid hormone medication should be taken at the same time each day to maintain constant hormone levels. **(M-S)**

▶ Thyroid hormone medication should be stored in tight, light-resistant bottles. **(M-S)**

▶ In Fowler's position, the head of the patient's bed is elevated 45 to 90 degrees. **(FND)**

▶ In semi-Fowler's or low Fowler's position, the head of the patient's bed is elevated 15 to 45 degrees. **(FND)**

▶ In high Fowler's position, the head of the patient's bed is elevated 90 degrees. **(FND)**

▶ A patient on nothing-by-mouth status can't receive ice chips to relieve dry mouth. **(FND)**

▶ A vasectomy doesn't affect a man's sexual potency, erections, or semen ejaculation. **(M-S)**

▶ The nurse who tells a patient, "Don't worry," "You look better and better every day," or "You'll be fine" is providing false reassurance. **(FND)**

▶ The nurse should use the ABCDE rule to prioritize nursing actions: Airway, Breathing, Circulation, Disease process, and Everything else. **(FND)**

▶ A retrospective audit is an evaluation of nursing care after it has been delivered. **(FND)**

▶ A concurrent audit is an evaluation of nursing care as it is being delivered. **(FND)**

▶ In a peer review, a nurse evaluates the work performed by a nurse of equal status. **(FND)**

▶ Desquamation is peeling of the skin. **(M-S)**

▶ When caring for the patient at risk for alcohol withdrawal, the nurse should monitor vital signs based on the patient's status. **(PSY)**

► Alcohol detoxification is most effective when it takes place in a structured environment with a supportive, nonjudgmental staff. **(PSY)**

► When caring for the patient experiencing alcohol withdrawal, the nurse should maintain a calm environment and minimize intrusions. **(PSY)**

► The alcoholic patient requires folic acid, oral thiamine, multivitamins, and adequate food and fluid intake. **(PSY)**

► The patient who is dependent on opiates typically has withdrawal symptoms within 12 hours after the last opiate dose. **(PSY)**

► The patient with Crohn's disease should consume a bland, low-residue diet that is high in proteins, calories, and vitamins. **(M-S)**

► Chronic carriers of hepatitis B test positive for hepatitis B surface antigen but are without signs of the disease. **(M-S)**

► Neurogenic bladder dysfunction results from conditions that affect bladder innervation. **(M-S)**

► Oxygen and carbon dioxide passively diffuse between alveoli and blood capillaries in the lungs. **(M-S)**

► When collecting 24-hour fractional urine specimens, the nurse should determine the number of bottles needed based on the time period. **(M-S)**

► A Logan bar is used postoperatively in the child recovering from cleft-lip repair. **(PED)**

► Aortic stenosis causes a loud, rough systolic murmur over the aortic area. **(M-S)**

► Required surgery is surgery that must be performed in the near future. **(M-S)**

► Urgent surgery is surgery that must be performed within 24 to 48 hours to prevent further harm to the patient. **(M-S)**

► Emergency surgery is surgery that must be performed immediately to save the patient's life. **(M-S)**

► Ambulatory surgery, often called outpatient or "in and out" surgery, requires no overnight stay in the hospital. **(M-S)**

► Urine has an acidic pH, normally around 6.0. **(M-S)**

► About 85% of arterial emboli originate from thrombi in the heart chambers. **(M-S)**

▶ When caring for the patient with an embolus in an arm or a leg, the nurse should keep the affected part at or below the horizontal plane. **(M-S)**

▶ Drug administration is a dependent function of the nurse. **(FND)**

▶ Jaundice arising during the first 24 hours after delivery signals erythroblastosis fetalis. **(MAT)**

▶ The nurse should instruct the outpatient to measure and record his pulse before taking verapamil. **(M-S)**

▶ The patient's urine is considered radioactive for 24 hours after radioisotope injection. **(M-S)**

▶ The nurse should teach the patient to take the oral antidiabetic drug chlorpropamide (Diabinese) in the morning. **(M-S)**

▶ Salivary amylase triggers starch digestion. **(M-S)**

▶ The patient experiencing pain from appendicitis should be placed in Fowler's position. **(M-S)**

▶ Analgesics can mask the pain of a ruptured appendix. **(M-S)**

▶ Nursing malpractice is negligence by the nurse that causes injury or harm to a patient. **(FND)**

▶ In true labor, the patient typically has pain and discomfort first in the back and then in the abdomen. **(MAT)**

▶ As a general rule, the nurse can't refuse a patient care assignment. **(FND)**

▶ To measure the height of the patient who can't stand, the nurse should mark the bed sheet at the top of the patient's head and at the bottom of the feet, and then measure the distance between the two marks. **(FND)**

▶ Esophageal perforation is suspected in the patient with an esophageal balloon tamponade if the patient complains of back pain or upper abdominal pain or if shock is present. **(M-S)**

▶ After reconstitution, a cephalosporin solution may change color if not used within 24 hours. **(M-S)**

▶ Chloramphenicol antagonizes the bactericidal action of penicillin. **(M-S)**

▶ A peripheral I.V. site should be changed every 48 to 72 hours. **(M-S)**

▶ During the early stage of shock, the patient's blood pressure may be normal but the respiratory and heart rates increase. **(M-S)**

▶ Cool, moist, pale skin, as occurs during shock, results from diversion of blood from the skin to major organs. **(M-S)**

▶ To assess capillary refill, the nurse should apply pressure over the nail bed until blanching occurs and then quickly release the pressure and note how quickly blanching fades (less than 3 seconds is normal). **(M-S)**

▶ The nursing process is a systematic, problem-solving method of providing nursing care. **(FND)**

▶ When giving an insulin injection, the nurse should use a 25G ⅝″ needle. **(M-S)**

▶ Residual urine (urine that remains in the bladder after voiding) normally measures 50 to 100 ml. **(M-S)**

▶ Assessment starts with the nurse's first encounter with the patient and continues throughout the health history interview and physical examination. **(FND)**

▶ During the planning stage of the nursing process, the nurse formulates and prioritizes nursing diagnoses, defines goals and expected outcomes, and develops the plan of care. **(FND)**

▶ During implementation, the nurse puts the plan of care into action, carrying out specific nursing actions and evaluating the patient's responses. **(FND)**

▶ During evaluation, the nurse determines whether the outcome criteria specified in the plan of care have been met and, if needed, modifies the plan. **(FND)**

▶ In the charting format known as "SOAP," S stands for subjective data, O for objective data, A for assessment data, and P for plans. **(FND)**

▶ In a SOAP note, subjective data consist of information obtained from the patient during the time elapsed since the last entry while objective data consist of physical findings and laboratory reports. **(FND)**

▶ The assessment (A) portion of a SOAP note includes evaluation of all data, etiology of the patient's problem, the course of the disease, and the patient's response to therapy. **(FND)**

▶ In a SOAP note, the plans (P) portion specifies what action to take, who should take it, and when it should be taken. **(FND)**

▶ The tonsils and adenoids serve as the first line of defense against respiratory infection. **(M-S)**

▶ A spermatozoon contributes either an X or a Y chromosome. **(MAT)**

▶ A miotic such as pilocarpine is used three to four times a day in a patient with glaucoma to cause pupillary constriction and to open the Schlemm's canal. **(M-S)**

▶ Weight gain is the most reliable indicator of a positive response to total parenteral nutrition therapy. **(M-S)**

▶ The nurse should suspect thrombophlebitis in the patient with Homans' sign. **(M-S)**

▶ When preparing the patient for a urinary catheterization, the nurse should place the female patient in the dorsal recumbent position with knees bent. **(M-S)**

▶ Metabolism has two phases—anabolism and catabolism. **(M-S)**

▶ Anabolism refers to metabolic reactions essential for growth and repair. **(M-S)**

▶ Catabolism refers to metabolic reactions that break down larger molecules to smaller ones to produce fuel for the body. **(M-S)**

▶ The most common cause of hyperthyroidism in the elderly is toxic nodular goiter. **(M-S)**

▶ The body processes foods in the following sequence: ingestion, digestion, absorption, transport, cell metabolism, and excretion. **(M-S)**

▶ Dietary fiber, or roughage, is derived from cellulose. **(M-S)**

▶ The body metabolizes alcohol at a fixed rate. **(M-S)**

▶ The alcohol concentration (proof) of a beverage indicates the percentage of alcohol multiplied by 2. **(M-S)**

▶ The liver metabolizes approximately 90% of ingested alcohol by using vitamin B to detoxify the alcohol. **(M-S)**

▶ Proteins make up the major portion of muscles, bones, skin, and hair. **(M-S)**

▶ Skinfold thickness reflects the amount of subcutaneous adipose tissue. **(M-S)**

▶ Red blood cells transport hemoglobin. **(FND)**

▶ White blood cells fight infection. **(FND)**

▶ Platelets form a hemostatic plug.   (FND)

▶ Hemophilia is an X-linked recessive bleeding disorder passed from the female to her male offspring.   (M-S)

▶ Von Willebrand's disease results from a platelet dysfunction and factor VIII deficiency and is more common in females than males.   (M-S)

▶ Sickle cell anemia is a chronic hemolytic anemia caused by hemoglobin S, a defective hemoglobin.   (M-S)

▶ Petechiae are tiny, round, red or purplish spots that may appear on the skin and mucous membranes.   (M-S)

▶ Purpura is a general term used to describe a purplish skin discoloration caused by extravasation of blood.   (M-S)

▶ Lavender-top tubes contain edetate, an anticoagulant; they are used to collect a sample of whole blood.   (M-S)

▶ Red-top tubes contain no additives; they are used to collect serum samples.   (M-S)

▶ Blue-top tubes contain sodium citrate and citric acid; they are used to collect plasma for coagulation studies.   (M-S)

▶ Grey-top tubes contain glycolytic inhibitor; they are usually used for serum glucose determination.   (M-S)

▶ Black-top tubes contain sodium oxalate; they are used to collect blood for coagulation studies.   (M-S)

▶ Green-top tubes contain heparin; they are used to collect serum samples for several studies.   (M-S)

▶ Heinz bodies in red blood cells indicate glucose-6-phosphate dehydrogenase deficiency.   (M-S)

▶ Patients usually receive a sedative 1 hour before a bone marrow biopsy.   (M-S)

▶ A butterfly rash on the bridge of the nose is a classic sign of systemic lupus erythematosus.   (M-S)

▶ A blood sample used for serum lithium measurement should be drawn immediately before the patient is to receive the next lithium dose, or 8 to 12 hours after the last dose was given.   (PSY)

▶ For an adult male, the normal daily caloric requirement is 2,300 to 3,100 calories.   (M-S)

▶ For an adult female, the normal daily caloric requirement is 1,600 to 2,400 calories. **(M-S)**

▶ Desensitization therapy, a process of slowly exposing the patient to a stimuli, is used to treat phobic disorders. **(PSY)**

▶ During nasotracheal suctioning, the nurse should maintain the infant's head in a neutral position by placing the infant on the back with a towel under the shoulders. **(PED)**

▶ The nurse should suction an infant for no more than 5 to 10 seconds at a time, pausing 1 to 3 minutes between each suctioning period. **(PED)**

▶ The umbilical cord is tied off approximately 1″ (2.5 cm) from the abdominal wall. **(MAT)**

▶ An ectopic pregnancy is an abnormal pregnancy in which the ovum implants outside the uterus. **(MAT)**

▶ The first stage of labor starts with the onset of contractions. **(MAT)**

▶ The second stage of labor ends with delivery of the infant. **(MAT)**

▶ The third stage of labor ends with placenta expulsion. **(MAT)**

▶ In a full-term neonate, the heel crease extends two-thirds of the way up the length of the heel; in a preterm neonate, the crease extends less than two-thirds. **(MAT)**

▶ Throughout pregnancy, a woman's blood volume increases but blood pressure should remain constant or slightly less. **(MAT)**

▶ Hegar's sign is a probable sign of pregnancy. **(MAT)**

▶ The multiparous woman is one who has given birth to one or more children. **(MAT)**

▶ The primigravida is a woman in her first pregnancy. **(MAT)**

▶ Goodell's sign is the softening of the cervix, a probable sign of pregnancy. **(MAT)**

▶ Melasma is a tan or brownish pigmentation on the face, especially the cheeks and nose, commonly seen in pregnant women. **(MAT)**

▶ Linea nigra often appears during pregnancy because of an increase in the hormone melatropin. **(MAT)**

▶ Presumptive signs of pregnancy are the least indicative signs of pregnancy and could indicate other conditions. **(MAT)**

▶ Probable signs of pregnancy can be documented by the examiner.
(MAT)

▶ Three fetal cardiac structures — the ductus venosus, foramen ovale, and ductus arteriosus — disappear after birth.   **(MAT)**

▶ The examiner can hear the fetal heartbeat with a Doppler device as early as the 10th to 12th week of pregnancy.   **(MAT)**

▶ At 12 to 14 weeks' gestation, the uterine fundus is palpable over the symphysis pubis and is considered an abdominal organ.   **(MAT)**

▶ At 36 weeks' gestation, the uterus is at the level of the xiphoid process.
(MAT)

▶ For a pelvic examination, the nurse should place the patient in the lithotomy position.   **(M-S)**

▶ Rubella poses the greatest risk to the embryo or fetus between the first 2 to 8 weeks of pregnancy.   **(MAT)**

▶ Live virus vaccines are contraindicated during pregnancy.   **(MAT)**

▶ Pregnant patients should avoid oral anticoagulants because these agents cross the placenta.   **(MAT)**

▶ Effleurage is a relaxation technique that can help distract the pregnant patient and reduce her pain.   **(MAT)**

▶ Spontaneous abortion and ectopic pregnancy are the most common causes of bleeding during the first trimester.   **(MAT)**

▶ The force of labor is supplied by the uterine fundus and implemented by uterine contractions.   **(MAT)**

▶ At 20 weeks' gestation, the uterine fundus should be at the level of the umbilicus.   **(MAT)**

▶ At 40 weeks' gestation, the uterine fundus is typically about 1½" (4 cm) below the xiphoid process (from lightening).   **(MAT)**

▶ The premature neonate is one whose gestational age is less than 38 weeks.   **(MAT)**

▶ The white line from the mons pubis to the umbilicus in the pregnant patient is referred to as linea alba.   **(MAT)**

▶ After the patient has a tonsillectomy, the nurse should suction out viscous mucus and provide warm saline gargles every 1 to 2 hours to relieve his pain, promote comfort, and help eliminate foul breath odor.   **(M-S)**

▶ The patient should be placed in a side-lying position immediately after surgery with an emesis basin to catch drainage and secretions until the patient is fully alert. **(M-S)**

▶ Bright red, moderate vaginal bleeding without cramping or cervical dilation signals a threatened abortion. **(MAT)**

▶ Complete abortion occurs when all products of conception have been expelled spontaneously without assistance. **(MAT)**

▶ Hydramnios is excessive amniotic fluid formation (more than 2,000 ml [67½ oz]). **(MAT)**

▶ Excessive vitamin K intake decreases the anticoagulant effect of warfarin (Coumadin). **(M-S)**

▶ After giving an I.M. injection, the nurse never should recap the needle and should discard it in an appropriate container. **(FND)**

▶ According to Freud, the genital stage of psychosexual development occurs from age 12 to 20. **(PED)**

▶ According to Erikson, the stage of identity versus confusion takes place from age 13 to 18. **(PED)**

▶ Tolerance means increasing resistance to the usual effects of a particular drug because of continued use. **(M-S)**

▶ The antidote for heparin is protamine sulfate. **(M-S)**

▶ The antidote for warfarin (Coumadin) is vitamin K. **(M-S)**

▶ A gallium scan may be used to detect primary or metastatic cancer. **(M-S)**

▶ On a child, mitt restraints should be removed at least twice each shift so the child can exercise his fingers. **(PED)**

▶ Bell's palsy results from inflammation of the seventh cranial nerve (the facial nerve). **(M-S)**

▶ In a nonreactive nonstress test, the fetal heart rate doesn't increase with fetal movement or fewer than five such responses occur in 20 minutes. **(MAT)**

▶ In a reactive nonstress test, the fetal heart rate increases by 15 beats/minute above the baseline in response to fetal activity, with five such responses occurring in 20 minutes. **(MAT)**

▶ The doctor may order a nonstress test for the pregnant patient with a prolonged pregnancy (over 41 weeks), diabetes, or a history of poor pregnancy outcomes or of intrauterine fetal death. **(MAT)**

► When feeding the infant who has a tracheostomy tube, the nurse should cover the opening with a moist gauze pad to prevent food or fluid from falling into the opening. **(PED)**

► When changing the ties on a tracheostomy tube, the nurse should leave the old ties in place until the new ones have been applied. **(M-S)**

► The nurse should always obtain help when changing the ties on an infant's tracheostomy tube. **(PED)**

► If an intradermal tuberculin skin test dose is injected too deeply, the nurse should inject another dose at a site 2″ (5 cm) away. **(M-S)**

► The intradermal tuberculin skin test should be read in 48 to 72 hours, when the induration is most evident. **(M-S)**

► Normal urine specific gravity measures 1.010 to 1.025. **(M-S)**

► When diagnosed early, cervical cancer has a cure rate of 95% to 100%. **(M-S)**

► Tuberculin skin tests are based on the principle of delayed hypersensitivity. **(M-S)**

► An example of a hypotonic solution is 0.33% sodium chloride solution. **(M-S)**

► Signs of hypernatremia include dry, sticky mucous membranes and a red, swollen tongue. **(M-S)**

► A pureed diet is commonly given to patients who have difficulty chewing or swallowing food. **(M-S)**

► The oxygen concentration of room air is 21%. **(M-S)**

► After a barium enema, the nurse should encourage the patient to drink more fluids to enhance barium elimination. **(M-S)**

► Proteinuria commonly indicates glomerular injury. **(M-S)**

► A delusion is a fixed false belief that persists and can't be corrected by reason. **(PSY)**

► An obstructed bile duct impairs absorption of nutrients and fat-soluble vitamins. **(M-S)**

► When mixing regular insulin with intermediate- or long-acting insulin, the nurse should draw the regular insulin into the syringe first. **(M-S)**

▶ After completing the assessment and nursing diagnosis steps of the nursing process, the nurse formulates desired goals (outcomes).
(FND)

▶ Assessing capillary refill is one way to check the circulatory status of a casted extremity. **(M-S)**

▶ When performing a venipuncture, the nurse first should select the most distal vein in the patient's hand, arm, leg, or foot. **(M-S)**

▶ All patients over age 65 should be assessed for aneurysm because of the normal vascular changes that accompany aging. **(M-S)**

▶ Tinnitus is a sign of salicylate (aspirin) toxicity. **(M-S)**

▶ Ulcers associated with Buerger's disease heal slowly. **(M-S)**

▶ Raynaud's disease is characterized by recurrent inflammation of the intermediate small veins of the extremities. **(M-S)**

▶ As Raynaud's disease progresses, the patient may develop ulcers and superficial gangrene of the hands. **(M-S)**

▶ OU denotes each eye or both eyes; OD denotes the right eye; and OS denotes the left eye. **(FND)**

▶ When removing a foreign body from the patient's eye, the nurse should irrigate with sterile normal saline solution. **(M-S)**

▶ For the patient with a corneal injury caused by a caustic substance, emergency care involves copious flushing of the eye with water.
(M-S)

▶ To remove an artificial eye, the nurse should pull down on the patient's lower lid and exert slight pressure on the eyelid to overcome suction holding the eye in place. **(FND)**

▶ The nurse should use normal saline solution to clean an artificial eye. **(FND)**

▶ Cataract surgery removes the lens of the patient's eye. **(M-S)**

▶ Severe pain after cataract surgery indicates increased intraocular pressure. **(M-S)**

▶ After ear irrigation, the nurse should place the patient on the affected side to allow any remaining fluid to drain. **(M-S)**

▶ Ascites is excess fluid in the peritoneal cavity. **(M-S)**

▶ A thready pulse is fine and scarcely perceptible. **(FND)**

▶ If the patient with an indwelling urinary catheter complains of abdominal discomfort, the nurse should check for bladder distention. **(M-S)**

▶ Bladder or urethral injury may result from an indwelling urinary catheter that is improperly positioned and secured.   **(M-S)**

▶ The nurse who accidentally inserts a urinary catheter into the patient's vagina should leave the catheter in place temporarily while starting the procedure over again using a new catheter.   **(M-S)**

▶ When assessing the patient with burns, the nurse should use the Rule of Nines to estimate burn extent and the percentage of body surface area burned.   **(M-S)**

▶ A partial-thickness burn involves the epidermis and part of the dermis.   **(M-S)**

▶ Taking the axillary temperature is the least accurate way of measuring body temperature.   **(FND)**

▶ After suctioning, the nurse must document the color, amount, consistency, and odor of secretions and the patient's tolerance for the procedure.   **(M-S)**

▶ "After meals" is abbreviated p.c.   **(FND)**

▶ After a bladder irrigation, the nurse should document the amount, color, clarity, and appearance of any clots or sediment in the urine.   **(M-S)**

▶ Semi-Fowler's position, diaphragmatic breathing, and relaxation are essential measures in the treatment of the patient having an asthma attack.   **(M-S)**

▶ Prostate cancer commonly metastasizes to the bone, lymph nodes, brain, and lungs.   **(M-S)**

▶ A needle's gauge indicates its diameter; the larger the gauge, the smaller the diameter.   **(FND)**

▶ After turning the patient, the nurse should document the position to which the patient was turned, the time of the turning, and skin assessment findings.   **(M-S)**

▶ In the patient with increasing intracranial pressure, the level of consciousness is the most significant indicator of health status.   **(M-S)**

▶ The acronym PERRLA means pupils equal, round, reactive to light, and accommodation.   **(FND)**

▶ When percussing the patient's chest during postural drainage, the nurse should cup her hands and percuss for 1½ to 2 minutes over each lobe. **(M-S)**

▶ Regular insulin is the only type of insulin that can be mixed with other insulins. **(M-S)**

▶ When taking the patient's radial pulse, the nurse should assess the rate, rhythm, quality, and force of the pulse. **(FND)**

▶ When documenting respirations, the nurse should include the rate, rhythm, depth, and quality. **(FND)**

▶ For a subcutaneous injection, the nurse should use a 25G ⅝" needle. **(FND)**

▶ The nurse should use passive range-of-motion exercises for the unconscious patient. **(M-S)**

▶ The nurse's notation "AA + O x 3" means the patient is awake and alert and oriented to person, place, and time. **(FND)**

▶ The respiratory center is located in the medulla oblongata. **(M-S)**

▶ Usually, foods and fluids are withheld for 8 hours before an I.V. pyelogram. **(M-S)**

▶ After giving an intradermal injection, the nurse shouldn't massage the injection site. **(FND)**

▶ When administering an intradermal injection, the nurse should hold the syringe almost parallel to the patient's skin, with the needle bevel up. **(FND)**

▶ The nurse should place a postthyroidectomy patient in semi-Fowler's position, with the head firmly supported by pillows (usually cervical pillows). **(M-S)**

▶ To obtain an accurate blood pressure, the nurse should pump the bulb until the mercury column or aneroid dial reaches 20 to 30 mm Hg above the point at which the pulse disappears or above the patient's baseline systolic pressure. **(FND)**

▶ Before giving castor oil to prepare the patient for a barium enema, the nurse may offer ice chips to minimize the bad taste. **(M-S)**

▶ If stoma color is much lighter than when last assessed, the nurse should suspect decreased circulation to the stoma. **(M-S)**

▶ In histrionic personality disorder, the patient displays manipulative behavior and dramatic emotional responses. **(PSY)**

► The nurse never should massage a leg with a blood clot because doing so may dislodge the clot. **(M-S)**

► Jaundice is commonly first detected by assessing the sclerae. **(M-S)**

► Jaundice results from a high serum bilirubin level. **(M-S)**

► Mydriatic drugs dilate the pupils. **(M-S)**

► Miotic drugs constrict the pupils. **(M-S)**

► After eye surgery, the nurse should place the patient on the unaffected side. **(M-S)**

► Infectious mononucleosis is called the "kissing disease" because it is transmitted by oral secretions. **(M-S)**

► The patient recovering from mononucleosis should stay in bed during periods of fever and should get additional rest at regular intervals. **(M-S)**

► Until recovery is complete, the patient with mononucleosis should avoid strenuous activity and competitive sports because the enlarged spleen is vulnerable to injury and may rupture from even mild trauma. **(M-S)**

► Skin traction applies direct pulling force to the skeleton and is most effective with children who have healthy skin tissue. **(M-S)**

► When placing a nitroglycerin patch on the patient, the nurse should avoid touching the medicated disk and wash her hands after application; gloves aren't required. **(M-S)**

► When caring for the patient with burns, the nurse should wear gloves, a gown, a mask, and protective headgear. **(M-S)**

► Before performing care procedures on the patient with burns, the nurse should administer prescribed pain medication. **(M-S)**

► The nurse should count an irregular pulse for 1 full minute. **(FND)**

► Black, tarry stools indicate upper GI tract bleeding. **(M-S)**

► The patient with a gastric ulcer should avoid aspirin and aspirin-containing products because they irritate the gastric mucosa. **(M-S)**

► If the patient starts to vomit while lying supine, the nurse should immediately place the patient on his side and maintain a patent airway. **(M-S)**

► A sitz bath usually lasts about 20 minutes. **(M-S)**

▶ The Apgar score is used to assess the neonate's vital functions; it is obtained 1 minute and 5 minutes after delivery. **(MAT)**

▶ After feeding the infant who has had surgery to repair a cleft lip or palate, the nurse should rinse the infant's mouth with sterile water. **(PED)**

▶ The infant who has undergone surgery to repair a cleft palate is at increased risk for otitis media. **(PED)**

▶ Surgical repair of a cleft palate is usually done when the infant is 4 to 6 months old and always before the child develops defective speech patterns. **(PED)**

▶ A cleft lip can be surgically corrected shortly after birth but may be delayed until the infant is 1 to 3 months old. **(PED)**

▶ When administering oral medication to the infant who has undergone cleft lip or palate surgery, the nurse should place the medication to one side of the mouth. **(PED)**

▶ Imaginative play is common in children around age 4. **(PED)**

▶ Negativism is characteristic of toddlers. **(PED)**

▶ The child with ascites caused by chronic liver disease should be placed in semi-Fowler's position. **(PED)**

▶ Autistic children fail to develop normal attachment behaviors. **(PED)**

▶ Toilet training is usually successful in toddlers. **(PED)**

▶ Applying erythromycin ointment to the neonate's eyes helps prevent gonorrheal conjunctivitis. **(MAT)**

▶ Gonorrhea rarely causes symptoms in adolescent females. **(M-S)**

▶ According to Erikson, the preschooler's developmental task is to gain initiative without experiencing guilt. **(PED)**

▶ Erythromycin ointment, used to prevent gonorrheal conjunctivitis in neonates, also eliminates chlamydia. **(M-S)**

▶ During the initial interview of the patient diagnosed with syphilis, the nurse should identify the patient's sexual contacts. **(M-S)**

▶ When suctioning the oral cavity and nasopharynx, the nurse should use a #5 to #8 French catheter in infants and a #8 to #10 French catheter in children. **(PED)**

▶ For nasotracheal suctioning, the nurse should set the suction regulator at 60 to 80 mm Hg for infants and 95 to 115 mm Hg for children. **(PED)**

▶ Remove any smoking material, such as matches, cigarettes, or cigars, from the room of the patient who is receiving oxygen and prominently place a "no smoking" sign in the room. **(M-S)**

▶ Flavoxate hydrochloride (Urispas) is used mainly as a urinary tract antispasmodic. **(M-S)**

▶ Signs and symptoms of cardiogenic shock result from loss of myocardial contractility, which causes reduced cardiac output. **(M-S)**

▶ Hypovolemic shock leads to an increased pulse, decreased systolic blood pressure, cold and clammy skin, pallor, thirst, an altered mental status, and decreased urine output. **(M-S)**

▶ Life-threatening arrhythmias are common during the first 24 hours after a myocardial infarction. **(M-S)**

▶ For the patient who has had a myocardial infarction, meticulous monitoring of fluid balance is crucial. **(M-S)**

▶ Cardiac output is determined by multiplying the stroke volume by the heart rate for 1 minute. **(M-S)**

▶ After a myocardial infarction, creatine kinase is the first enzyme level to increase. **(M-S)**

▶ The nurse should use normal saline solution to irrigate a nasogastric tube. **(M-S)**

▶ If the patient with a nasogastric tube complains of a sore nostril, the nurse should apply a water-soluble lubricant. **(M-S)**

▶ The nurse may give anesthetic lozenges or use gargles to relieve a sore throat caused by irritation from the nasogastric tube. **(M-S)**

▶ During the first 12 to 24 hours after gastric surgery, suctioned stomach contents appear brown. **(M-S)**

▶ The lactate dehydrogenase level rises within 12 hours after the onset of a myocardial infarction. **(M-S)**

▶ After a myocardial infarction, cardiac enzyme levels rise; the higher they rise and the longer they remain at peak levels, the more serious the heart muscle damage. **(M-S)**

▶ The nurse should use low intermittent suction when suctioning a nasogastric tube. **(M-S)**

▶ When documenting drainage on a surgical dressing, the nurse should chart the amount, color, and consistency of drainage. **(M-S)**

▶ In rare instances, electroconvulsive therapy has caused arrhythmias and even death. **(PSY)**

▶ Confusion and memory loss are among the most common mental status changes after electroconvulsive therapy. **(PSY)**

▶ Classic signs of pyloric stenosis are a palpable olive-sized mass in the right upper abdominal quadrant, visible strong peristalsis moving left to right after feeding, and projectile vomiting. **(PED)**

▶ Valvular venous insufficiency is the most likely cause of varicose veins. **(M-S)**

▶ The patient with a colostomy should restrict intake of fatty and fibrous foods and should avoid foods that can obstruct the stoma. **(M-S)**

▶ During chemotherapy, the patient with a depressed white blood cell count is placed on neutropenic precautions. **(M-S)**

▶ The patient with mitral valve stenosis typically has signs and symptoms associated with improper emptying of the left atrium and subsequent pulmonary congestion. **(M-S)**

▶ Mitral valve stenosis usually arises as a complication of rheumatic fever. **(M-S)**

▶ If a chest tube gets disconnected, the nurse should clamp it immediately. **(M-S)**

▶ Atelectasis is an abnormal condition characterized by collapse of lung tissue and incomplete expansion of lobules (clusters of alveoli) or a lung segment. **(M-S)**

▶ To perform cardiopulmonary resuscitation, the nurse should place the victim on a flat, solid surface. **(M-S)**

▶ Antacids interfere with absorption of histamine-receptor antagonists. **(M-S)**

▶ The patient with an ileal conduit should empty the collection device before it is half full. **(M-S)**

▶ To assess a patient for a distended bladder, the nurse should check for a rounded mass above the pubis. **(M-S)**

▶ To test for Babinski's reflex, the nurse should firmly stroke the lateral aspect of the patient's sole. In a positive response, the patient dorsiflexes the big toe and extends and fans the other toes. **(M-S)**

▶ A positive human immunodeficiency virus test indicates the patient has been infected with the virus that causes acquired immunodeficiency syndrome. **(M-S)**

▶ Because human immunodeficiency virus appears in breast milk, it can be transmitted by breast-feeding. **(MAT)**

▶ For the patient with heart failure, decreasing the heart's workload is one of the nurse's primary goals. **(M-S)**

▶ Performing meticulous skin care and turning the bedridden patient every 2 hours are the most effective ways to prevent skin breakdown. **(M-S)**

▶ The nurse should suspect an asthma attack in the patient who wheezes, coughs, or exhibits respiratory distress. **(M-S)**

▶ The nurse should advise the patient with an ileostomy to eat foods that deodorize the GI tract, such as spinach and parsley. **(M-S)**

▶ After an adrenalectomy, decreased steroid production may lead to extensive loss of sodium and water. **(M-S)**

▶ During the first 24 hours after delivery, many women have a low-grade fever, which results from dehydration caused by labor. **(MAT)**

▶ Antiembolism stockings provide gradual compression of the superficial blood vessels, helping to prevent thrombus formation. **(M-S)**

▶ The patient who no longer requires bed rest after a femoral-popliteal bypass graft should be permitted to walk and stand. **(M-S)**

▶ The nurse should record ice chips as fluid intake at approximately half their volume. **(M-S)**

▶ Of the five senses, hearing is thought to be the last sense lost by comatose patients. **(M-S)**

▶ In an adult, the most convenient veins for venipuncture are the basilic and median cubital veins. **(M-S)**

▶ The drug zidovudine (AZT) is used to prevent replication of human immunodeficiency virus. **(M-S)**

▶ *Pneumocystis carinii* pneumonia is an opportunistic infection associated with acquired immunodeficiency syndrome. **(M-S)**

▶ If a radioactive implant becomes dislodged, the nurse should retrieve the device with tongs and place it in a lead-shielded container. **(M-S)**

▶ The patient receiving external radiation therapy should pat the skin dry. **(M-S)**

▶ The nurse should give aluminum hydroxide separately and at least 1 hour apart from enteric-coated medications. **(M-S)**

▶ By age 12 months, the infant has typically tripled his birth weight and has eight teeth. **(PED)**

▶ Acid-base balance is the body's hydrogen ion concentration. **(M-S)**

▶ Buffers are substances in the blood that prevent body fluid from becoming overly acidic or alkaline. **(M-S)**

▶ Metabolic acidosis results from excessive bicarbonate loss or excessive production or retention of acid. **(M-S)**

▶ In homonymous hemianopsia, blindness occurs in half the patient's visual field in one or both eyes. **(M-S)**

▶ Full weight bearing is restricted for 3 to 6 months following a total hip replacement. **(M-S)**

▶ After a total knee replacement, the doctor determines how soon the patient is allowed to bear weight. **(M-S)**

▶ Before giving an intermittent tube feeding, the nurse should verify correct tube placement. **(M-S)**

▶ People with type O blood are known as universal donors. **(FND)**

▶ People with type AB blood are known as universal recipients. **(FND)**

▶ Nausea, vomiting, restlessness, and twitching are signs of disequilibrium syndrome resulting from rapid fluid shift. **(M-S)**

▶ In "setting sun," a sign of increased intracranial pressure, the iris is displaced downward and the sclera appears above the iris. **(PED)**

▶ Electroconvulsive therapy is most effective in treating patients with severe depression. **(PSY)**

▶ For electroconvulsive therapy to be effective, the patient should receive a total of 6 to 12 treatments; usually, two or three treatments are given per week. **(PSY)**

▶ Return of reflex activity in the extremities below the injury level indicates that spinal shock is resolving. **(M-S)**

▶ When caring for the patient with stomatitis, the nurse should provide frequent mouth care. **(M-S)**

▶ Hearing protection is required when sound intensity increases above 84 decibels. **(M-S)**

▶ In otitis media, the patient typically has a bright red tympanic membrane and an absent light reflex (cone of light). **(M-S)**

▶ In pericardiocentesis, blood is withdrawn from the pericardial sac. **(M-S)**

▶ During labor, the resting phase between each contraction should last at least 30 seconds. **(MAT)**

▶ Urticaria is one of the first signs of a hemolytic transfusion reaction. **(M-S)**

▶ During peritoneal dialysis, return of brown dialysate indicates bowel perforation. **(M-S)**

▶ Early signs and symptoms of ketoacidosis include polyuria, polyphagia, fatigue, malaise, drowsiness, headache, and abdominal pain. **(M-S)**

▶ In the infant with hydrocephalus, a high-pitched cry signals increasing intracranial pressure. **(PED)**

▶ Prothrombin, a clotting factor, is produced by the liver. **(M-S)**

▶ If the patient is menstruating when a urine sample is collected, the nurse should note this on the laboratory slip. **(M-S)**

▶ During a lumbar puncture, the patient should refrain from holding his breath to prevent interfering with pressure readings. **(M-S)**

▶ The rash associated with scarlet fever starts 12 to 48 hours after onset of pharyngeal symptoms. **(M-S)**

▶ The recommended adult dose of sucralfate (Carafate) is 1 g (1 tablet) four times a day, taken on an empty stomach. **(M-S)**

▶ Lochia rubra is the vaginal discharge that occurs during the first 3 days postpartum. **(MAT)**

▶ Lochia serosa is the serous pink or brown vaginal discharge that appears from days 3 to 7 postpartum. **(MAT)**

▶ Lochia alba is the white discharge occurring from days 7 to 10 postpartum; it may last up to 6 weeks. **(MAT)**

▶ The patient should have nothing by mouth after midnight on the day before any surgery involving general anesthesia. **(M-S)**

▶ The patient who has inhaled smoke should be hospitalized for 24 hours to allow observation for delayed tracheal edema. **(M-S)**

▶ After a burn, two stages of physiologic changes occur: the hypovolemic stage and the diuretic stage. **(M-S)**

▶ When administering total parenteral nutrition, the nurse should change the tubing at least every 24 hours and should change the dressing over the insertion site every 72 hours. **(M-S)**

▶ The nurse should store total parenteral nutrition solutions in a refrigerator and remove them 1 hour before administration. **(M-S)**

▶ Colostrum is the thin, yellow fluid secreted by the breasts during pregnancy and the first postpartum days before lactation starts. **(MAT)**

▶ From a prepregnancy length of about 2½″ (6.5 cm), the uterus grows to about 12½″ (32 cm) at term. **(MAT)**

▶ The pelvis's diagonal conjugate diameter, which can be measured directly, is used to estimate the true conjugate diameter. **(MAT)**

▶ Fetal heart tones are the most reliable indicator of fetal status. **(MAT)**

▶ The nurse should use standard precautions when caring for the patient with tuberculosis. **(M-S)**

▶ When performing pin care for the patient in skeletal traction, the nurse's highest priority is to prevent osteomyelitis. **(M-S)**

▶ For the patient with carbon monoxide poisoning, the nurse should administer humidified oxygen, as ordered, until the carboxyhemoglobin level measures less than 5%. **(M-S)**

▶ The sweat chloride test is used to confirm a diagnosis of cystic fibrosis. **(PED)**

▶ The nurse should avoid giving routine I.M. injections into edematous tissue because the medication may not be absorbed. **(M-S)**

▶ In the patient receiving dialysis, a palpated thrill or an auscultated bruit indicates that the internal shunt is working. **(M-S)**

▶ Early signs of acquired immunodeficiency syndrome include flulike symptoms, such as fatigue, night sweats, enlarged lymph nodes, anorexia, weight loss, pallor, and fever. **(M-S)**

▶ Late decelerations of the fetal heart rate indicate uteroplacental insufficiency. **(MAT)**

▶ During the manic phase of bipolar affective disorder, the nurse should protect the patient from self-injury or exhaustion.   **(PSY)**

▶ To control the rapid emergence of the fetus's head during an emergency delivery, the nurse should place a hand on the head of the fetus and apply only enough pressure to guide the descent.   **(MAT)**

▶ Multiparous patients are at greater risk for postpartum bleeding than primiparous patients.   **(MAT)**

▶ Safety measures are the primary concern for the nurse caring for the patient with Alzheimer's disease.   **(M-S)**

▶ The patient is usually the best source of health history information.   **(FND)**

▶ The patient with Parkinson's disease usually receives levodopa (Dopar) to compensate for dopamine deficiency.   **(M-S)**

▶ Patients with multiple sclerosis are at increased risk for pressure ulcers.   **(M-S)**

▶ Palliative therapy is used to relieve or reduce symptoms; it doesn't produce a cure.   **(M-S)**

▶ Pill-rolling tremors are a classic sign of Parkinson's disease. **(M-S)**

▶ A primary nursing goal for the patient with Parkinson's disease is to improve mobility and help the patient gain independence in self-care.   **(M-S)**

▶ Blood urea nitrogen normally measures 10 to 20 mg/dl.   **(M-S)**

▶ Metrorrhagia — vaginal bleeding between menstrual periods — may be the first sign of cervical cancer.   **(M-S)**

▶ When caring for the comatose patient, the nurse should explain each step to the patient in a normal voice.   **(M-S)**

▶ The patient receiving phenytoin sodium (Dilantin) is at risk for gingival hyperplasia.   **(M-S)**

▶ When providing denture care, the nurse should line the sink with a washcloth or a paper towel to prevent denture breakage if they are dropped.   **(M-S)**

▶ The patient should void within 6 to 8 hours after surgery.   **(M-S)**

▶ EEG identifies normal and abnormal brain waves.   **(M-S)**

▶ Migraine headaches cause persistent, severe pain — usually in the temporal region.   **(M-S)**

▶ The patient in a bladder retraining program should void every 2 hours during the day and twice at night. **(M-S)**

▶ The cardiovascular and respiratory systems are regulated by the autonomic nervous system. **(M-S)**

▶ Ergotamine tartrate (Ergostat) is an effective treatment for migraine or vascular headaches. **(M-S)**

▶ Signs and symptoms of hiatal hernia include fullness in the upper abdominal region, heartburn, and reflux. **(M-S)**

▶ Prophylaxis refers to disease prevention. **(M-S)**

▶ Women who have borne children have a higher incidence of cholelithiasis than any other group. **(M-S)**

▶ Ascites and jaundice are prominent signs of advanced liver disease. **(M-S)**

▶ Obstipation is protracted constipation or the absence of bowel movements. **(M-S)**

▶ Roasted chicken, rice, and pound cake are appropriate foods for the patient on a low-residue diet. **(M-S)**

▶ A rectal tube should remain in place for 20 to 30 minutes. **(M-S)**

▶ Trust is the foundation of the nurse-patient relationship. **(FND)**

▶ Proper body alignment means that body parts are in correct relationship to their natural anatomical position. **(M-S)**

▶ For the postoperative patient, a diet high in carbohydrates and proteins is most therapeutic. **(M-S)**

▶ Blood pressure reflects the pressure exerted on the arterial walls as blood is forced through them. **(FND)**

▶ Patients with hepatitis B should be instructed never to donate blood. **(M-S)**

▶ Patients undergoing radiation therapy should protect their skin markings because they are landmarks for treatment. **(M-S)**

▶ A biopsy and cytological examination of the tumor specimen provide the most definitive diagnosis of cancer. **(M-S)**

▶ Patients in methadone maintenance programs should receive methadone dissolved in 4 oz (120 ml) of orange juice or a powdered citrus drink unless the drug is provided in a liquid form. **(PSY)**

▶ Joint repair is called arthroplasty. **(M-S)**

▶ When giving a bed bath, the nurse should clean the patient in this sequence: face, neck, arms, hands, chest, abdomen, back, legs, and perineum. **(FND)**

▶ To avoid self-injury when lifting and moving a patient, the nurse should use the large muscles of her thighs. **(FND)**

▶ A malignant tumor of connective tissue is called a sarcoma. **(M-S)**

▶ Subluxation is a partial dislocation of a joint. **(M-S)**

▶ Aluminum hydroxide (Amphojel) decreases gastric acidity. **(M-S)**

▶ Barbiturates may cause confusion and delirium in elderly patients with organic brain disorders. **(PSY)**

▶ Physical therapy promotes optimal functioning in the patient with arthritis. **(M-S)**

▶ Most patients with hepatitis A are anicteric (lacking jaundice). **(M-S)**

▶ Adding a toe pleat to the top sheet makes a patient's feet more comfortable. **(FND)**

▶ Hepatitis A is highly contagious during the preicteric phase. **(M-S)**

▶ The nurse must follow standard precautions when caring for a patient with hepatitis A. **(M-S)**

▶ Cholecystography isn't effective in diagnosing the patient with gallstones because the stones may obstruct the cystic duct and prevent the contrast medium from entering the gallbladder. **(M-S)**

▶ Anticipatory grief is grief that arises in anticipation of an inevitable death or significant loss. **(M-S)**

▶ Because of polyuria, dehydration is a major concern for patients with diabetes insipidus. **(M-S)**

▶ To guard against a charge of malpractice, the nurse should provide care in a reasonable and prudent manner. **(FND)**

▶ The patient may receive methohexital sodium (Brevital), a general anesthetic, before an electroconvulsive therapy treatment. **(PSY)**

▶ Maintaining a patent airway is the nurse's highest priority when caring for the patient receiving an electroconvulsive therapy treatment. **(PSY)**

▶ The decision to use restraints on the patient must be based on safety. **(M-S)**

▶ The doctor may prescribe diphenhydramine hydrochloride (Benadryl) to relieve extrapyramidal adverse reactions of psychotropic medications. **(PSY)**

▶ The patient stabilized on lithium should have blood drug levels drawn every month. **(PSY)**

▶ To prevent "purple glove" syndrome, the nurse shouldn't administer phenytoin I.V. through a vein in the back of the patient's hand. **(M-S)**

▶ Psychotropic medications are used to relieve symptoms and allow the patient to participate in therapy. **(PSY)**

▶ Through behavior, the manipulative patient is asking to be controlled. **(PSY)**

▶ The patient with signs or symptoms of lithium toxicity should be instructed not to take any additional doses and to be examined by a doctor. **(PSY)**

▶ Alcoholics Anonymous teaches members that untreated chemical dependency is progressive. **(PSY)**

▶ Methylphenidate hydrochloride (Ritalin) is the drug of choice for children with attention deficit hyperactivity disorders. **(PED)**

▶ Setting consistent limits is the most effective way to control a patient's manipulative behavior. **(PSY)**

▶ Violent outbursts are common in patients with borderline personality disorder. **(PSY)**

▶ When caring for the depressed patient, the nurse should explore meaningful losses. **(PSY)**

▶ An illusion is a false interpretation of a sensory stimulus. **(PSY)**

▶ Extrapyramidal adverse reactions are common in patients taking antipsychotic medications. **(PSY)**

▶ Anxiety is a vague sense of impending doom or apprehension without real cause. **(PSY)**

▶ Signs and symptoms of Cushing's syndrome result mainly from unregulated secretion of glucocorticoids and androgens. **(M-S)**

▶ Confabulation is a speech pattern and is the unconscious filling in of memory gaps with fabricated information. **(PSY)**

▶ The goal of any therapy is to bring about a positive change. **(PSY)**

▶ Catharsis is the therapeutic release of pent-up feelings and emotions by open discussion of ideas and thoughts. **(PSY)**

▶ A basic assumption of psychoanalytic theory is that all behavior has a cause and can be explained. **(PSY)**

▶ Total parenteral nutrition solutions contain glucose, amino acids, and electrolytes. **(M-S)**

▶ Regional anesthesia may involve the use of topical anesthetics, local infiltration, nerve blocks, or subdural or epidural blocks. **(M-S)**

▶ Children between ages 2 and 3 discover masturbation as an enjoyable activity while exploring their bodies. **(PED)**

▶ Respiratory paralysis occurs during stage IV of general anesthesia. **(M-S)**

▶ The nurse should encourage ambulation in the postpartum patient who complains of gas pains and flatulence. **(MAT)**

▶ After placenta delivery, uterine massage helps to stimulate contractions. **(MAT)**

▶ During phototherapy, the nurse should cover the infant's eyes to prevent retinal injury. **(MAT)**

▶ Crackles indicate lung congestion caused by fluid or pus. **(M-S)**

▶ Bronchovesicular breath sounds are abnormal when heard over the peripheral lung fields. **(M-S)**

▶ Wheezing is an abnormal, high-pitched breath sound that indicates obstruction or closure of the bronchi. **(FND)**

▶ The nurse should use mineral oil to remove an insect from the patient's external ear canal. **(M-S)**

▶ If the patient complains that a hearing aid isn't working, the nurse should first check the switch and batteries. **(M-S)**

▶ The nurse should grade hyperactive deep tendon reflexes with sustained clonus as +4. **(FND)**

▶ Vertigo is the major assessment finding in the patient with Ménière's disease. **(M-S)**

▶ The nurse should instruct the patient with an upper respiratory infection to blow his nose with both nostrils open. **(M-S)**

▶ The infant with gastroesophageal reflux should receive formula thickened with cereal. **(PED)**

▶ A patient can resume most normal activities 3 or 4 days after cataract surgery. **(M-S)**

▶ Ocular irritation, a decreasing visual field, corneal edema, and scleral redness are signs of corneal transplant graft rejection. **(M-S)**

▶ A child should visit the dentist by age 2. **(PED)**

▶ Wisdom teeth commonly appear between ages 17 and 21. **(PED)**

▶ Signs and symptoms of Graves' disease include nervousness, irritability, weight loss, palpitations, increased thirst, and exophthalmos. **(M-S)**

▶ When caring for the postoperative patient who is allowed to have oral intake, the nurse should force fluids to help prevent constipation. **(M-S)**

▶ Preschoolers don't view death as final, but do fear separation from their parents. **(PED)**

▶ Portals of exit for infection transmission include the mouth, nose, feces, urine, vomitus, blood, and vaginal and penile discharge. **(M-S)**

▶ Breech presentation of the fetus increases the risk of a prolapsed umbilical cord, fetal head trauma, and fracture of the fetal spine or arm. **(MAT)**

▶ A nasal cannula delivers oxygen concentrations of 22% to 44%. **(M-S)**

▶ Postmenopausal women receiving estrogen replacement therapy are at increased risk for gallbladder disease. **(M-S)**

▶ The hormone oxytocin stimulates powerful uterine contractions during labor. **(MAT)**

▶ Prolactin stimulates breast milk production. **(MAT)**

▶ Diabetes insipidus is manifested by polyuria and polyphagia. **(M-S)**

▶ The patient with diabetic ketoacidosis experiences osmotic diuresis leading to dehydration and electrolyte loss. **(M-S)**

▶ Cushing's syndrome causes moon face, buffalo hump, acne, mood swings, hirsutism, amenorrhea, and a decreased libido. **(M-S)**

▶ In group therapy, each member of the group gets an opportunity to examine interactions, learn and practice successful interpersonal communication skills, and explore emotional conflicts. **(PSY)**

▶ Signs of a nasal fracture include internal and external bleeding, swelling of adjacent soft tissues, and deformity. **(M-S)**

▶ The nurse should elevate the head of the bed when caring for the patient with heart failure. **(M-S)**

▶ Lip cancer causes a painless, indurated ulcer with raised edges. **(M-S)**

▶ The patient whose signs and symptoms suggest cerebrovascular accident should be placed on the affected side. **(M-S)**

▶ After chest surgery, the nurse should encourage the patient to frequently raise the arm on the affected side above the head. **(M-S)**

▶ Variable decelerations of the fetal heart rate indicate umbilical cord compression or prolapse. **(MAT)**

▶ Mitosis has four phases: (1) prophase, (2) metaphase, (3) anaphase, and (4) telophase. **(M-S)**

▶ The nurse should withhold all preparations containing vitamin D from the patient receiving calcifediol (Calderol). **(M-S)**

▶ In the patient receiving digoxin, a below-normal serum potassium level increases the risk of digitalis toxicity. **(M-S)**

▶ The patient with diabetes insipidus may crave cold water. **(M-S)**

▶ Flurazepam (Dalmane) toxicity causes mental confusion, hallucinations, and ataxia. **(M-S)**

▶ A "silent" myocardial infarction causes no symptoms. **(M-S)**

▶ Adverse effects of verapamil (Calan) include dizziness, headache, constipation, hypotension, and atrioventricular conduction disturbances. **(M-S)**

▶ Yellowish-green wound drainage indicates an infection. **(M-S)**

▶ During a sickle cell crisis, severe pain in the hands and feet is known as "hand-foot" syndrome. **(M-S)**

▶ Oral candidiasis causes white plaques with a milk-curd appearance on the oral mucosa, gums, or tongue. **(M-S)**

▶ The patient with paranoid personality disorder displays pervasive and long-standing suspicions reflecting a lack of basic trust. **(PSY)**

▶ The person with antisocial personality disorder perceives others and the world in general as hostile and harmful. **(PSY)**

▶ Failing to provide a safe, secure environment for a child constitutes child neglect. **(FND)**

▶ The most common psychiatric disorder is depression. **(PSY)**

▶ Cytomegalovirus, a member of the herpesvirus family, can cause extensive fetal damage. **(MAT)**

▶ Infants with cerebral palsy may display asymmetrical movements, difficulty feeding, and an excessive or feeble cry. **(PED)**

▶ Anorexia, weight loss, abdominal pain, and jaundice may be the first signs and symptoms of pancreatic cancer. **(M-S)**

▶ Adverse effects of tricyclic antidepressant drugs may include tachycardia and orthostatic hypotension. **(PSY)**

▶ Tocolytic therapy typically is indicated for the patient in premature labor. **(MAT)**

▶ Snow blindness is a temporary dimming of vision caused by the glare of the sun on snow. **(M-S)**

▶ Hodgkin's disease characteristically causes a painless, progressive enlargement of lymph nodes. **(M-S)**

▶ In Huntington's chorea, degeneration of the cerebral cortex and basal ganglia results in progressive dyskinetic movements and mental deterioration. **(M-S)**

▶ The nurse should stay alert for suicidal behavior in patients with Huntington's chorea. **(M-S)**

▶ Foods high in vitamin D include fortified milk, fish, liver, liver oil, herring, and egg yolk. **(M-S)**

▶ For a pelvic examination, the nurse should place the patient in the lithotomy position. If the patient can't assume a lithotomy position (for example, because of advanced age or poor health), the nurse should place her on her left side. **(M-S)**

▶ During a vaginal examination, a female assistant should be present if the examiner is male. **(M-S)**

▶ Before ovulation, the cervical mucus is thick and doesn't stretch when pulled between the thumb and finger. **(M-S)**

▶ Body fluid discoloration is a common adverse effect of rifampin (Rimactane). **(M-S)**

▶ Liver function studies should be done before a patient starts isoniazid (INH) therapy. **(M-S)**

► Bread and cereal are good sources of thiamine, iron, niacin, and riboflavin. **(M-S)**

► Central cyanosis is the most significant sign of hypoxia. **(M-S)**

► "Good Samaritan Laws" protect professionals who provide assistance at the scene of an emergency without fear of a lawsuit arising from such assistance. **(FND)**

► Within 24 hours, the doctor should sign medical orders given verbally or by telephone. **(FND)**

► The nurse should refer the patient's questions regarding informed consent to the doctor. **(FND)**

► The competent adult has the right to refuse life-saving medical treatment; however, the patient must be fully informed of the consequences of refusal. **(FND)**

► The intoxicated patient isn't considered competent for the purposes of refusing required medical treatment. **(FND)**

► The patient's health record or chart is the hospital's physical property; however, the contents belong to the patient. **(FND)**

► The patient or legal guardian must give written consent before the patient's records can be released to a third party. **(FND)**

► The nurse can't perform duties that violate a rule or regulation established by a state licensing board. **(FND)**

► When caring for the hostile or angry patient, the nurse should try to remain calm and continue to listen without showing disapproval. **(FND)**

► When caring for the sick or injured child with limited communication skills, the nurse may encourage the child to draw pictures expressing his feelings. **(PED)**

► To conduct the health history interview, the nurse should choose a private room, preferably one with a door that can be closed. **(FND)**

► When caring for the acutely ill or agitated patient, the nurse should limit questions to those that could provide essential information. **(FND)**

► The nurse should wait 15 minutes after the patient has smoked a cigarette or taken anything by mouth before taking his temperature orally. **(FND)**

► The nurse shouldn't use her thumb to take the patient's pulse. **(FND)**

▶ When counting respirations, the nurse should count an inspiration and expiration as one respiration. **(FND)**

▶ Kussmaul's respiration is a breathing pattern in which respirations are abnormally fast and deep and aren't separated by pauses. **(FND)**

▶ In Cheyne-Stokes respiration, periods of deep, rapid breathing alternate with periods of apnea. **(FND)**

▶ Eupnea is normal respiration. **(FND)**

▶ Biot's respiration is characterized by periods of apnea alternating with periods in which the patient takes four or five breaths of identical depth. **(FND)**

▶ Before thyroid surgery, hyperthyroid patients usually receive potassium iodine to reduce goiter size and vascularity. **(M-S)**

▶ When taking blood pressure, the nurse should support the patient's arm rather than letting the patient use his own strength to hold the arm up. **(FND)**

▶ Nonmodifiable risk factors for coronary artery disease include heredity, sex, race, and age. **(M-S)**

▶ Inspection is the most frequently used assessment technique. **(FND)**

▶ The nurse should instruct the pregnant vegetarian patient to obtain adequate protein from nonmeat sources. **(MAT)**

▶ The pregnant patient should take only prescribed prenatal vitamins and should avoid high-potency, over-the-counter "megavitamin" preparations. **(MAT)**

▶ Foods high in sodium can cause fluid retention. **(M-S)**

▶ Adding fiber to the diet can help the pregnant patient avoid constipation and hemorrhoids. **(M-S)**

▶ The normal life cycle of a red blood cell is 120 days. **(M-S)**

▶ Ritualism is a typical behavior in a toddler. **(PED)**

▶ The person with 20/100 vision sees at 20′ (6.1 m) what a person with normal vision sees at 100′ (30.5 m). **(M-S)**

▶ According to Freud's psychosexual theory, the oral stage occurs from birth to age 18 months. **(PED)**

▶ Food interferes with penicillin absorption. **(M-S)**

▶ Offering a favorite "chaser," such as orange juice, is one way to get the child to swallow oral medication. **(PED)**

▶ To provide a "homey" atmosphere, the nurse should advise family members to transfer personal items when moving the patient to a skilled nursing facility. **(FND)**

▶ When prioritizing nursing diagnoses, the nurse should give life-threatening problems top priority. **(FND)**

▶ When developing the nursing plan of care, the nurse should write patient outcomes in measurable, observable terms, along with target dates for their completion. The acronym SMART means specific, measurable, achievable, reasonable, time factor. **(FND)**

▶ Spinal shock is loss of all spinal reflexes and sensations below the injury level after spinal cord transection. **(M-S)**

▶ When inserting a nasogastric tube, the nurse should aim the tube downward and toward the ear that is closer to the chosen nostril. **(M-S)**

▶ The nurse should inform the patient taking oral iron (ferrous sulfate) that the preparation may turn stools dark green to black. **(M-S)**

▶ Polycythemia vera causes pruritus, pain in the fingers and toes, hyperuricemia, a florid complexion, weakness, and easy fatigue. **(M-S)**

▶ Rheumatic fever is usually preceded by a group A beta-hemolytic streptococcal infection. **(M-S)**

▶ Thyroid storm is a medical crisis caused by uncontrolled hyperthyroidism. **(M-S)**

▶ Tardive dyskinesia causes involuntary repetitive movements of the face and mouth, such as lip smacking, and can progress to other abnormal movements. **(M-S)**

▶ Vision is usually fully developed by age 7. **(PED)**

▶ The nurse shouldn't give raisins, hot dogs, or round foods to an infant because these foods may cause choking. **(PED)**

▶ Hydrocephalus is the most common complication of surgical closure of a myelomeningocele. **(PED)**

▶ In the patient with hemophilia, repeated hemorrhages may cause degenerative joint changes, osteoporosis, and muscle atrophy. **(M-S)**

▶ For the child with failure to thrive, the goal of care is to promote an age-appropriate growth and development pattern. **(PED)**

▶ The patient with mania should avoid competitive games, heated group discussions, and excessive physical exercise. **(PSY)**

▶ After a thyroidectomy, hoarseness or a whispery voice suggests laryngeal nerve damage. **(M-S)**

▶ After intracranial surgery, the nurse should keep the patient in a lateral or semiprone position until consciousness returns. **(M-S)**

▶ During the immediate postoperative period after intracranial surgery, the nurse should monitor the patient's vital signs and assess level of consciousness for signs of increasing intracranial pressure. **(M-S)**

▶ Techniques used in chest physiotherapy include percussion (patting the back with cupped hands) and vibration (placing the hands over the affected area and vigorously quivering them). **(M-S)**

▶ Folic acid and vitamin B_{12} are essential for nucleoprotein synthesis and red blood cell maturation. **(M-S)**

▶ The nurse should encourage the parents of a hearing-impaired child to communicate through mime, gestures, and body language. **(PED)**

▶ Patients receiving prednisone should consume a high-protein, high-potassium, low-salt diet. **(M-S)**

▶ As a general rule, neonates require 120 cal/kg of body weight at birth. **(MAT)**

▶ Clues suggesting physical abuse of a child include a parent's implausible explanation of how the child's injuries occurred. **(PED)**

▶ In geriatric patients, age-related changes and multiple medications contribute to a high incidence of noncompliance with drug therapy. **(M-S)**

▶ "Strawberry tongue" is a sign of Kawasaki disease. **(M-S)**

▶ A first-degree burn involves the stratum corneum, the skin's outermost layer; it causes pain and reddened skin. **(M-S)**

▶ The patient being treated for an asthma attack should be placed in semi- to high-Fowler's position depending on the patient's comfort. **(M-S)**

▶ Tuberculosis is a reportable communicable disease caused by *Mycobacterium tuberculosis*, an acid-fast bacillus. **(M-S)**

▶ In right-sided cardiac catheterization, a radiopaque catheter passes through the antecubital or femoral vein into the patient's right atrium, right ventricle, and pulmonary vasculature. **(M-S)**

▶ The average length of the menstruation cycle is 28 days.   **(M-S)**

▶ McDonald's rule is used to measure fundal height.   **(MAT)**

▶ Nägele's rule (subtract 3 months from the first day of the last menstrual period and then add 7 days) is used to calculate the expected date of delivery.   **(MAT)**

▶ Amenorrhea is a presumptive sign of pregnancy.   **(MAT)**

▶ The nurse should inform the pregnant patient that oral sex during pregnancy may cause air embolism.   **(MAT)**

▶ Human chorionic gonadotropin in the blood or urine is a probable sign of pregnancy.   **(MAT)**

▶ The pregnant woman should avoid exposure to X-rays, especially during the first trimester.   **(MAT)**

▶ Sexual intercourse during pregnancy is contraindicated if the amniotic membranes have ruptured or vaginal bleeding has occurred.   **(MAT)**

▶ Milia are small papules sometimes seen on the cheek or the bridge of the nose in neonates.   **(MAT)**

▶ The union of the male and female gamete results in a zygote. **(MAT)**

▶ In a cerebrovascular accident, blood vessels in the brain are blocked by an embolus or hemorrhage, resulting in decreased blood supply to brain tissues normally perfused by the damaged vessels.   **(M-S)**

▶ After a fracture, a bone heals in the following sequence: inflammation, cellular proliferation, callus formation, ossification, and remodeling.   **(M-S)**

▶ The nurse shouldn't administer atropine sulfate to the patient with glaucoma.   **(M-S)**

▶ Once the zygote becomes implanted in the uterus, it is called an embryo.   **(FND)**

▶ Fetal growth occurs in a cephalocaudal fashion.   **(FND)**

▶ The pons is located in front of the cerebellum, between the midbrain and medulla.   **(M-S)**

▶ Smooth muscles are controlled by the autonomic nervous system.   **(M-S)**

▶ The patient who sits in a wheelchair too long may develop flexion contractures of the hips.   **(M-S)**

▶ Immediate care for a sprain or strain consists of applying ice and elevating the limb above the level of the patient's heart. **(M-S)**

▶ According to Erikson, the main conflict of the young adult (ages 19 to 35) is intimacy versus isolation. **(FND)**

▶ Erikson proposed that the main conflict of the older adult (ages 65 and older) is integrity versus despair. **(FND)**

▶ Family therapy focuses on the family as a whole rather than the individual member. **(PSY)**

▶ The erythrocyte sedimentation rate normally measures 0 to 15 mm/hour for males under age 50 and 0 to 20 mm/hour for females under age 50. **(M-S)**

▶ In culdoscopy, the doctor visualizes the pelvic organs using an endoscope inserted through the posterior vaginal wall. **(M-S)**

▶ Propranolol (Inderal) blocks the sympathetic nerve stimulation that increases the cardiac workload during exercise or stress. **(M-S)**

▶ Electrocardiogram changes usually appear during the first 24 hours after a myocardial infarction. However, in some cases, they are delayed for 5 to 6 days. **(M-S)**

▶ Cottage cheese, fish, canned beans, chuck steak, chocolate pudding, Italian salad dressing, dill pickles, and beef broth are extremely high in sodium. **(M-S)**

▶ Dried prunes, watermelon, dried lima beans, soybeans, bananas, and oranges are high in potassium. **(M-S)**

▶ The neonate of a diabetic mother should be assessed for hypoglycemia. **(MAT)**

▶ The patient who has delivered a stillborn child should be allowed to hold the child to help her come to terms with the death. **(MAT)**

▶ An infant develops the concept of object permanence by age 6 to 10 months. **(PED)**

▶ During the sensorimotor stage, a child begins to learn about cause-and-effect relationships. **(PED)**

▶ According to Erikson, a child begins to develop a conscience during the preschool years (ages 3 to 6). **(FND)**

▶ Molding is the shaping of the fetal head as it adjusts to the shape and size of the birth canal. **(MAT)**

▶ Liver dysfunction may cause difficulty metabolizing certain drugs.
(M-S)

▶ The nurse should monitor the patient's blood pressure closely if a pudendal block is administered before delivery. **(MAT)**

▶ If the patient suddenly becomes hypotensive during labor, the nurse should increase the flow rate of I.V. fluids, as ordered. **(MAT)**

▶ After placenta delivery, the nurse should anticipate adding oxytocin to the I.V. solution. **(MAT)**

▶ Early deceleration of the fetal heart rate results from fetal head compression during uterine contractions, and no treatment is indicated. **(MAT)**

▶ Pregnant patients should take folic acid because this nutrient is essential for rapid cell division. **(MAT)**

▶ In such conditions as burns and malnutrition, edema results from a decrease in capillary osmotic pressure. **(M-S)**

▶ Fluid volume deficit is a potential complication of nasogastric suctioning. **(M-S)**

▶ Pulmonary congestion may lead to fluid accumulation throughout the body. **(M-S)**

▶ The woman with a spinal cord injury may be able to become pregnant. **(M-S)**

▶ During the first few days after onset of intracranial bleeding, nursing care should focus on providing a quiet, restful environment.
(M-S)

▶ The patient receiving clomiphene citrate (Clomid) to induce ovulation should be told that this drug may cause multiple gestation.
(M-S)

▶ A slapping gait and blindness are associated with neurosyphilis.
(M-S)

▶ Increasing intracranial pressure is the most serious complication of a cerebrovascular accident. **(M-S)**

▶ The pregnant patient with an incompetent cervix usually undergoes cervical suturing between weeks 14 and 18 to help her maintain the pregnancy. **(MAT)**

▶ To pinpoint the bleeding site in the patient with an intracranial hemorrhage, the doctor may order a cerebral arteriogram. **(M-S)**

▶ Factors affecting drug action include drug absorption, distribution, metabolism, and excretion. **(M-S)**

▶ During the first trimester of pregnancy, the patient should refrain from taking any drug unless lack of drug therapy would adversely affect her health. **(MAT)**

▶ Before a drug is prescribed to a woman of childbearing age, the physician should rule out the possibility of pregnancy. **(M-S)**

▶ Most drugs ingested by a lactating woman appear in her breast milk. **(MAT)**

▶ Patients with glucose-6-phosphate dehydrogenase deficiency may develop hemolytic anemia when given sulfonamides. **(M-S)**

▶ Acidosis may cause insulin resistance. **(M-S)**

▶ The five pregnancy risk categories (A, B, C, D, and X) identify a drug's potential risk to the fetus. **(M-S)**

▶ The nurse should use the bell of the stethoscope to listen for venous hums and murmurs. **(FND)**

▶ The chief complaint is a subjective statement made by the patient describing his most significant needs and concerns. **(FND)**

▶ Turner's sign (also called Grey-Turner's sign) is seen in patients with acute pancreatitis. **(M-S)**

▶ The patient with a gastric ulcer typically complains of gnawing or burning epigastric pain. **(M-S)**

▶ To assess the patient's general knowledge level and orientation, the nurse should ask such questions as "Who is the president of the United States?". **(FND)**

▶ The first cranial nerve is the olfactory nerve. **(M-S)**

▶ The patient with cerebellar disease has an ataxic gait. **(M-S)**

▶ To check for cerebrospinal fluid leakage, the nurse should inspect the patient's nose and ears for leakage. **(M-S)**

▶ Reye's syndrome is associated with aspirin use after certain viral illnesses such as chickenpox. **(M-S)**

▶ Compression syndrome occurs when pressure caused by edema pushes against encased arteries, veins, and nerves. **(M-S)**

▶ The patient with a ruptured ectopic pregnancy typically complains of sharp pain in the lower abdomen, along with spotting and cramping. **(MAT)**

▶ The nurse should warn the patient receiving prednisone or another steroid not to stop taking the drug abruptly. **(M-S)**

▶ Alanine aminotransferase and aspartate aminotransferase are liver enzymes. **(M-S)**

▶ The normal serum calcium level measures 4.5 to 5.5 mEq/L. **(M-S)**

▶ The normal serum sodium level ranges from 135 to 145 mEq/L. **(M-S)**

▶ The normal serum potassium level measures 3.5 to 5.0 mEq/L. **(M-S)**

▶ The patient on continuous ambulatory peritoneal dialysis must use sterile technique when performing catheter care. **(M-S)**

▶ The Minnesota Multiphasic Personality Inventory is an objective test used to assess personality traits and characteristic ego responses to stress. **(PSY)**

▶ The Stanford-Binet test assesses the intelligence and cognitive abilities of children under age 16. **(PED)**

▶ T cells are involved in the cell-mediated immune response. **(M-S)**

▶ For infants at high risk for acquired immunodeficiency syndrome, positive antibody results are considered reliable after age 15 months. **(PED)**

▶ When caring for the patient with acquired immunodeficiency syndrome, the nurse should wear a mask and protective eyewear if splashes of blood or other body fluids are likely to occur. **(M-S)**

▶ The cardinal movements of labor are descent, flexion, internal rotation, extension, external rotation, and expulsion. **(MAT)**

▶ Bence-Jones protein is used to confirm the diagnosis of multiple myeloma. **(M-S)**

▶ Gaucher's disease is an autosomal disorder characterized by abnormal accumulation of glucocerebrosides. **(M-S)**

▶ The patient with a colon obstruction usually complains of lower abdominal pain, constipation, increasing abdominal distention, and vomiting. **(M-S)**

▶ Currant-jelly stools are a sign of intussusception. **(M-S)**

▶ D.S. added to the name of a drug means "double strength." **(FND)**

▶ Allopurinol (Lopurin) is used to prevent or treat attacks of gout.
(M-S)

▶ Uric acid is an end product of purine metabolism. **(M-S)**

▶ The normal sperm count is 120 to 300 million/ml. **(M-S)**

▶ The man with a sperm count below 60 million/ml is considered infertile. **(M-S)**

▶ The most common psychiatric disorder seen in a mental health setting is depression. **(PSY)**

▶ If the patient's uterus is boggy after placenta delivery, the nurse should firmly massage the fundus. **(MAT)**

▶ Passage of flatus and the return of bowel sounds indicate resumption of gastric motility. **(M-S)**

▶ A person may use defense mechanisms to protect the ego during periods of anxiety. **(PSY)**

▶ *Projection* refers to an unconscious defense mechanism in which the person displaces generally negative feelings onto another individual. **(PSY)**

▶ In the defense mechanism called *displacement*, the person transfers an emotion from its original object to a substitute. **(PSY)**

▶ The child with attention deficit hyperactivity disorder commonly has difficulty learning. **(PSY)**

▶ The person with agoraphobia is afraid of being alone or in a public area from which escape would be difficult or help would be unavailable in the event of suddenly becoming disabled. **(PSY)**

▶ *Dementia* refers to a progressive organic mental disorder characterized by memory and intellectual deficits, disorientation, and decreased cognitive function. **(PSY)**

▶ The white blood cell count normally ranges from 4,000 to 10,000/μl. **(M-S)**

▶ Serum cholesterol levels of 200 to 320 mg/dl are considered above normal. **(M-S)**

▶ Serum thyroxine (T_4) levels normally measure 5 to 13.5 mcg/dl. **(M-S)**

▶ Production of human chorionic gonadotropin peaks around the 10th week of gestation. **(MAT)**

▶ Port wine-colored amniotic fluid may indicate abruptio placentae.
(MAT)

▶ A lecithin-sphingomyelin ratio above 2:1 indicates fetal lung maturity.
(MAT)

▶ A chorionic villi sampling is used to detect fetal chromosomal abnormalities.
(MAT)

▶ Cloudy cerebrospinal fluid indicates infection. **(M-S)**

▶ During a lumbar puncture, crying, coughing, or straining may increase cerebrospinal fluid.
(M-S)

▶ To determine how far to insert a nasogastric tube, the nurse should measure the distance from the tip of the patient's nose to the earlobe and then add this measurement to the measured distance from the earlobe to the base of the xiphoid process. **(FND)**

▶ After a colonoscopy, signs and symptoms of bowel perforation include malaise, rectal bleeding, abdominal pain and distention, fever, and mucopurulent drainage. **(M-S)**

▶ A *tort* is a wrongful act committed outside of a contractual relationship. **(FND)**

▶ *Slander* refers to a false and defamatory oral statement about a person. **(FND)**

▶ Careful, accurate, and complete documentation is the nurse's best protection against a lawsuit. **(FND)**

▶ In Maslow's hierarchy of needs, physiologic needs are the most basic, followed in descending order by safety and security, belonging and affection, esteem and self-respect, and self-actualization. **(FND)**

▶ According to Maslow, primary needs must be met to maintain life; secondary needs must be met to maintain the quality of life. **(FND)**

▶ The first teeth are called the *deciduous* teeth. **(PED)**

▶ Abstinence is the only method that is 100% effective in preventing pregnancy and sexually transmitted diseases. **(M-S)**

▶ The mother can nurse the newborn immediately after birth. **(MAT)**

▶ *Ossification* refers to the development of bone. **(M-S)**

▶ Cranial nerve II (the optic nerve) is a sensory nerve responsible for vision. **(M-S)**

▶ The patient with schizophrenia commonly has an absent, flat, blunted, or inappropriate affect. **(PSY)**

▶ Crisis intervention focuses only on the patient's immediate problems. **(PSY)**

▶ Quality assurance in health care refers to evaluation of services provided and the results achieved as compared to accepted standards; such evaluation typically includes the quality, quantity, appropriateness, and costs of health services provided. **(FND)**

▶ All patients have the right to considerate and respectful care. **(FND)**

▶ *Beneficence* refers to the quality or state of producing good, such as performing acts of charity or kindness. **(FND)**

▶ The geriatric patient normally has decreased bladder capacity and a delayed voiding sensation. **(M-S)**

▶ In patients with Alzheimer's disease, death typically results from a complication. **(M-S)**

▶ The serum glucose level normally ranges from 70 to 110 mg/dl. **(M-S)**

▶ Lactated Ringer's solution is an isotonic solution. **(M-S)**

▶ A serum sodium level below 135 mEq/L indicates hyponatremia. **(M-S)**

▶ The nurse shouldn't use a cotton-tipped applicator to dry the patient's ear canal or to remove wax. **(FND)**

▶ The nurse should instruct the patient with a history of heat stroke to wear loose-fitting clothing, rest frequently, and drink plenty of fluids. **(FND)**

▶ All central venous catheter ports should be capped when not in use. **(M-S)**

▶ An EEG identifies normal and abnormal brain waves. **(M-S)**

▶ Signs and symptoms of premenstrual syndrome include abdominal distention, engorged and painful breasts, backache, headache, and irritability. **(M-S)**

▶ A hip fracture is the most common fracture type in geriatric patients. **(M-S)**

▶ During a continuous tube feeding, the nurse should irrigate the tube every 6 hours. **(M-S)**

▶ The GI tract isn't sterile. **(M-S)**

▶ In an adult, hypothyroidism may cause coarse, dry hair with patchy hair loss or thinning. **(M-S)**

▶ A hair comb should have dull teeth, as opposed to sharp teeth that could injure the patient. **(FND)**

▶ Hypothermia refers to a below-normal body temperature. **(FND)**

▶ Tepid water measures 80° to 98° F (27° to 37° C). **(FND)**

▶ When using a heat lamp, the nurse should direct the lamp to the side of the treatment area, not directly over it. **(FND)**

▶ Foods that become liquid at room temperature or break down into liquid in the GI tract must be charted as fluid intake. **(FND)**

▶ One unit of blood contains 500 ml. **(FND)**

▶ The nurse should administer routine medications within 30 minutes of the ordered time. **(FND)**

▶ Heparin is the drug of choice for treatment of thromboembolic disease. **(M-S)**

▶ The surgeon can extract an embolus from a large artery using a Fogarty embolectomy catheter. **(M-S)**

▶ Blockage of a large artery by an embolus is a life-threatening emergency that necessitates surgery. **(M-S)**

▶ Acute iliofemoral venous thrombosis causes limb enlargement; it can be detected by measuring the affected part and comparing it to the opposite extremity. **(M-S)**

▶ The areas that sustain the greatest damage from arteriosclerosis are the brain, heart, GI tract, kidneys, and extremities. **(M-S)**

▶ The nurse should inform the patient receiving phenazopyridine (Pyridium) that this drug colors the urine orange or red. **(M-S)**

▶ To obtain the child's rectal temperature, the nurse should insert the thermometer only 1″ (2.5 cm) into the rectum. **(PED)**

▶ Normally, the neonate's urine specific gravity measures 1.002 to 1.010 after ingesting milk. **(PED)**

▶ Laboratory test results are considered objective data. **(FND)**

▶ *Pneumocystis carinii* pneumonia usually causes disease only in people with suppressed immune systems. **(M-S)**

▶ For best absorption, patients should take erythromycin tablets with a full glass of water 1 hour before or 2 hours after a meal. **(M-S)**

▶ *Trismus* is a sign of tetanus. **(M-S)**

▶ Operating room nurses generally are held liable for failing to keep an accurate count of sponges and other items used in surgery. **(M-S)**

▶ Defense mechanisms protect the personality by reducing stress and anxiety. **(PSY)**

▶ *Suppression* is the conscious inhibition of thoughts that provoke stress or anxiety. **(PSY)**

▶ Warfarin sodium (Coumadin) is an oral anticoagulant. **(M-S)**

▶ Infants should be weighed and measured monthly until at least age 6 months. **(PED)**

▶ During the oral phase (the first 18 months), the infant derives satisfaction and pleasure from sucking and chewing. **(PED)**

▶ Infancy lasts from birth to age 12 months. **(PED)**

▶ The toddler stage starts at age 1 and ends at age 3. **(PED)**

▶ The patient at risk for a pressure ulcer shouldn't be placed on a trochanter (a 30-degree lateral position is recommended) when the side-lying position is used. **(FND)**

▶ Foods high in iron include organ meats, nuts, legumes, dried fruits, leafy vegetables, eggs, and whole grains. **(FND)**

▶ The best sources of vitamin B_6 are liver, kidney, muscle meats, soybeans, corn, and whole-grain cereals. **(FND)**

▶ For a thoracentesis, the nurse should position the patient upright, if possible. **(M-S)**

▶ Blood not transfused within 30 minutes after it's obtained should be returned to the blood bank. **(FND)**

▶ To administer a blood transfusion, the nurse should hang the blood bag 3′ to 4′ above the level of the patient's heart. **(FND)**

▶ Gas bubbles and discoloration in a blood bag indicate bacterial growth. **(M-S)**

▶ Before transfusing a large amount of blood, the nurse should use a warming coil to warm it to a temperature above 98.7° F (37° C). **(M-S)**

▶ A breast-feeding woman can clean each nipple with a cotton ball and sterile water, using a circular motion. **(MAT)**

▶ Initially, the neonate should breast-feed for 2 to 5 minutes at each breast and then progress gradually to breast-feeding for 10 or 15 minutes every 2 to 3 hours. **(MAT)**

▶ To ease tender skin on the breasts or nipples, a breast-feeding woman should use only a mild emollient cream prescribed by the doctor. **(MAT)**

▶ Breast-feeding women should increase their daily fluid intake by 500 to 900 ml. **(MAT)**

▶ The nurse should place the patient with a closed chest drainage system in semi-Fowler's position and encourage hourly coughing by manual splinting of the chest. **(M-S)**

▶ In a one-bottle closed drainage system, the bottle acts as a water seal, providing suction and drainage collection; therefore, it shouldn't be emptied. **(M-S)**

▶ In a two-bottle closed chest drainage system, the first bottle collects drainage while the second acts as a water seal and controls suction. **(M-S)**

▶ In a three-bottle closed chest drainage system, the first bottle collects drainage, the second acts as a water seal, and the third controls suction. **(M-S)**

▶ During colostomy irrigation, the nurse should hang the irrigating bag 18″ to 20″ above the stoma. **(M-S)**

▶ The temperature of fluid used for colostomy irrigation shouldn't exceed 105° F (40.5° C). **(M-S)**

▶ Signs of an arterial obstruction caused by an embolism include absent pulse, anesthesia, paralysis, and pale, cool skin. **(M-S)**

▶ Hyperventilation is associated with respiratory alkalosis. **(M-S)**

▶ A mineral oil enema is contraindicated for patients with appendicitis, an acute surgical abdomen, fecal impaction, or intestinal obstruction. **(M-S)**

▶ Psychodrama is used in group therapy to help participants gain new perceptions and self-awareness. **(PSY)**

▶ The patient involuntarily admitted to a psychiatric hospital doesn't have the right to sign out against medical advice. **(PSY)**

▶ "People who live in glass houses shouldn't throw stones" and "A rolling stone gathers no moss" are examples of proverbs that may be used during a psychiatric interview to evaluate the patient's abstract reasoning ability. **(PSY)**

▶ Before carrying out a nursing procedure for a patient, the nurse should go by this rule: Always assess before action. **(FND)**

▶ Case management nursing involves a case manager who plans and coordinates patient care activities. **(FND)**

▶ Pinpoint pupils are a sign of acute narcotic intoxication. **(M-S)**

▶ The nursing history consists mainly of subjective assessment data. **(FND)**

▶ The physical examination provides objective assessment data obtained by using the senses. **(FND)**

▶ The nurse gathers objective assessment data through inspection, percussion, palpation, and auscultation. **(FND)**

▶ Diagnostic test results provide objective assessment data. **(FND)**

▶ The patient's toenails can be cleaned with an orangewood stick while his foot is immersed in water. **(FND)**

▶ A complete nursing diagnosis consists of the patient problem, the etiology (cause or contributing factor) of the problem, and any signs or symptoms that help to clarify the nursing diagnosis. **(FND)**

▶ The patient's nails should be clipped and filed straight across, even with the end of the digit. **(FND)**

▶ The nurse should categorize nursing diagnoses by priority. **(FND)**

▶ Signs and symptoms of acute barbiturate intoxication may resemble those of alcohol intoxication. **(M-S)**

▶ A labile affect is characterized by a rapid shift of emotions and mood. **(PSY)**

▶ *Amnesia* refers to memory loss resulting from an organic or inorganic cause. **(PSY)**

▶ Borderline personality disorder is marked by pervasive instability of self-image, mood, and interpersonal relationships. **(PSY)**

▶ Decreased renal function makes geriatric patients more susceptible to dehydration. **(M-S)**

▶ The nurse should use a shorter needle when giving an I.M. injection to the elderly patient. **(FND)**

▶ *Stress incontinence* is intermittent urine leakage resulting from a sudden increase in intra-abdominal pressure, such as from coughing, laughing, or running. **(M-S)**

▶ The heart has four valves: tricuspid, mitral, pulmonic, and aortic. **(M-S)**

▶ The patient in restraints should be checked every 15 to 30 minutes; each restraint should be removed every 2 hours. **(FND)**

▶ The patient on disulfiram (Antabuse) shouldn't receive metronidazole (Flagyl) because the two drugs may interact to cause a psychotic reaction. **(M-S)**

▶ *Urge incontinence* is the inability to control a sudden urge to urinate. **(M-S)**

▶ *Total incontinence* is continued urine leakage. **(M-S)**

▶ Elderly people commonly suffer constipation because of reduced intestinal motility. **(M-S)**

▶ Protein, vitamin, and mineral needs usually remain constant as a person ages. **(FND)**

▶ The elderly patient grows shorter as the intervertebral spaces narrow and the spinal curvature increases. **(M-S)**

▶ When converting grams to grains, the nurse should remember the following rule: 1 g = 1,000 mg = 15 gr. **(FND)**

▶ Before giving informed consent, the patient must receive information that would affect a reasonable person's decision to consent to or refuse a treatment or procedure, including a description of the treatment or procedure, its potential risks and adverse effects, and possible effects of not having the treatment or procedure. **(FND)**

▶ The patient must sign a separate informed consent form for each treatment or procedure. **(FND)**

▶ Gout progresses in four stages: (1) asymptomatic hyperuricemia, (2) acute gouty arthritis, (3) intercritical gout, and (4) chronic tophaceous gout. **(M-S)**

▶ The nursing plan of care includes the nursing diagnosis, expected outcomes (or goals), nursing interventions, and evaluation criteria. **(FND)**

▶ If the patient received a sedative before signing an informed consent, the nurse should promptly notify the appropriate doctor. **(FND)**

▶ During the acute phase of gout, the nurse should use a bed cradle to raise the sheets and blankets off the patient's sensitive joints. **(M-S)**

▶ The spouse of the patient who's a minor may give permission for the patient to undergo a treatment or procedure. **(FND)**

▶ Congenital hip dysplasia is the most common hip joint disorder in children younger than age 3. **(PED)**

▶ Heparin inactivates thromboplastin and thrombin. **(M-S)**

▶ Placing a familiar object or picture on a door may assist the confused patient in finding his room without help. **(PSY)**

▶ The patient is demonstrating autonomy when making a decision about the time he will take a bath. **(M-S)**

▶ For the patient with traction pins, preventing infection is the main purpose of providing skin care. **(M-S)**

▶ The patient receiving morphine shouldn't receive anticholinesterase agents because the resulting drug interaction may cause respiratory depression. **(M-S)**

▶ The main purpose of play therapy is to allow the child to express feelings and frustrations. **(PED)**

▶ *Reframing* provides the patient with alternative ways of viewing a situation. **(PSY)**

▶ The early stage of Alzheimer's disease is manifested by short-term memory loss. **(PSY)**

▶ Profound changes in personal relationships occur during the middle to advanced stages of Alzheimer's disease. **(PSY)**

▶ During the final stage of Alzheimer's disease, total memory loss occurs. **(PSY)**

▶ The nurse should wash her hands with warm, not hot, water; warm water removes fewer protective skin oils. **(FND)**

▶ The cause of essential hypertension is unknown. **(M-S)**

▶ Administration of propranolol (Inderal) reduces portal pressure and decreases the risk of bleeding from esophageal varices. **(M-S)**

▶ The nurse should administer sedatives with caution to a patient with cirrhosis. **(M-S)**

▶ The patient whose burn wound is infected with *Staphylococcus aureus* must be kept in strict isolation. **(M-S)**

▶ The patient undergoing external radiation therapy should be instructed to avoid applying creams or lotions to the treatment site. **(M-S)**

▶ Strabismus is a normal finding in the neonate. **(MAT)**

▶ The most common vascular complication of diabetes mellitus is atherosclerosis. **(M-S)**

▶ Insulin deficiency may lead to hyperglycemia. **(M-S)**

▶ Drooling, a masklike expression, pill rolling, and a propulsive gait are signs of Parkinson's disease. **(M-S)**

▶ The point of maximal impulse is located at the fifth intercostal space near the heart apex. **(FND)**

▶ The first heart sound (S_1) represents closure of the mitral and tricuspid valves. **(FND)**

▶ The second heart sound (S_2) represents closure of the aortic and pulmonic valves. **(FND)**

▶ Threatening the patient with an injection for failing to take an oral medication is considered assault. **(FND)**

▶ The coronary artery supplies blood to the myocardium. **(M-S)**

▶ The patient with gouty arthritis should increase his fluid intake to prevent renal calculi formation. **(M-S)**

▶ The nurse should instruct the patient on a low-salt diet to avoid canned vegetables. **(FND)**

▶ The patient receiving furosemide (Lasix) should eat bananas and citrus fruits because they're a good source of potassium. **(M-S)**

▶ Dyspnea is a common sign of left ventricular failure. **(M-S)**

▶ The nurse should encourage the patient at risk for pneumonia to turn frequently, cough, and deep-breathe. **(M-S)**

▶ If the patient's blood pressure rises above baseline, the nurse should notify the doctor. **(FND)**

▶ Buck's traction is used to immobilize and reduce spasms before surgery in the patient with a fractured hip. **(FND)**

▶ When caring for the patient with a fractured hip, the nurse should check the neurovascular status of extremities every 2 hours. **(M-S)**

▶ The nurse should use an abduction pillow or trochanter rolls to maintain abduction in the postoperative patient with a fractured hip. **(FND)**

▶ A fiberglass cast is more durable and dries faster than a plaster cast. **(M-S)**

▶ In the immobilized patient, the most important circulatory complication to watch for is pulmonary embolism. **(M-S)**

▶ To relieve edema associated with an extremity fracture, the nurse should elevate the affected limb. **(M-S)**

▶ The treatment of choice for the patient with osteomyelitis is I.V. antibiotics. **(M-S)**

▶ The postpartum patient may resume sexual intercourse after perineal and uterine wounds have healed (usually 2 to 6 weeks after delivery). **(MAT)**

▶ The pregnant nurse shouldn't be assigned to work with a patient infected with cytomegalovirus. **(MAT)**

▶ The nurse should suspect abuse if the patient's wounds are inconsistent with the stated history or if various wounds are in different stages of healing. **(FND)**

▶ Respiratory distress syndrome is common in premature neonates. **(MAT)**

▶ *Fetal demise* refers to death of the fetus after the age of viability (considered to be 20 weeks). **(MAT)**

▶ Administering oxytocin (Pitocin) is the most commonly used method for inducing labor after artificial rupture of the membranes. **(MAT)**

▶ Ensuring comfort is the nurse's highest priority when caring for the terminally ill patient. **(M-S)**

▶ The patient prone to constipation should increase dietary bulk. **(M-S)**

▶ Dorsiflexion is recommended for immediate relief of leg cramps. **(M-S)**

▶ After cardiac surgery, the patient should be placed on a diet that provides 2 g of sodium and 300 mg of cholesterol. **(M-S)**

▶ After the amniotic membranes rupture, the nurse's top priority is monitoring the fetal heart rate. **(MAT)**

▶ Bleeding after intercourse is an early sign of cervical cancer. **(M-S)**

▶ Oral hypoglycemics stimulate insulin secretion from the pancreatic islet cells. **(M-S)**

▶ Use of drugs such as antibiotics is a common cause of vaginal infections. **(M-S)**

▶ The kidneys play a major role in maintaining the body's fluid balance. **(M-S)**

▶ People visiting the patient with a radiation implant must limit their stay to 10 minutes. **(M-S)**

▶ Reexamining one's goals is a major developmental task during middle adulthood. **(FND)**

▶ Docusate sodium (Colace) helps prevent straining during defecation. **(M-S)**

▶ Headache and restlessness are early indicators of delirium tremens. **(PSY)**

▶ According to most experts, the acute stage of alcohol detoxification encompasses the first 72 hours after consumption ends. **(PSY)**

▶ After prostatic surgery, the primary cause of pain is the indwelling urinary catheter. **(M-S)**

▶ The pregnant woman who has a cat is at increased risk for toxoplasmosis. **(MAT)**

▶ Telangiectatic nevi ("stork bites") are flat red or purple lesions that may appear on the neonate's nose, upper eyelids, or the back of the neck. **(MAT)**

▶ When assessing the neonate after a breech birth, the nurse should check for brachial nerve palsy. **(MAT)**

▶ Spontaneous abortion is a possible complication of amniocentesis. **(MAT)**

▶ If the pregnant patient's urine tests positive for acetone but negative for glucose, her diet must be assessed for adequate protein intake. **(MAT)**

▶ During pregnancy, lack of exercise or a calcium deficiency may cause leg cramps. **(MAT)**

▶ Orange juice and green vegetables are good sources of folic acid. **(FND)**

▷ Rubella exposure during pregnancy is associated with fetal heart defects. **(MAT)**

▷ When using the Glasgow Coma Scale, the nurse assesses the patient's verbal response, motor response, and eye openings. **(FND)**

▷ During the first 24 hours after a major burn, the patient should receive nothing by mouth and should receive I.V. fluid replacement according to the Brooke or Evans formula. **(M-S)**

▷ The nurse should place an unconscious patient in low Fowler's position when administering an intermittent nasogastric tube feeding. **(M-S)**

▷ *Decorticate positioning* refers to an abnormal posture in which the patient's arms are adducted (toward the core of the body) and flexed, with the wrists and fingers flexed on the chest. **(M-S)**

▷ When caring for the patient with drug-induced psychosis, the nurse should find out when the drug was taken to help determine if it can be evacuated from the patient's body. **(M-S)**

▷ The patient with a condition that may necessitate surgery should receive nothing by mouth until cleared by the doctor. **(M-S)**

▷ During the first trimester of pregnancy, increased hormonal levels may cause nausea and vomiting. **(MAT)**

▷ Meperidine (Demerol) may be used to relieve the pain of nephrolithiasis. **(M-S)**

▷ The nurse should institute measures to protect the patient with thrombocytopenia from injury. **(M-S)**

▷ Immediately after the patient dies, the nurse should place the body in a normal position. **(FND)**

▷ Trendelenburg's test, which evaluates venous filling, is used to check for incompetent valves in the patient with varicose veins. **(M-S)**

▷ *Decerebrate positioning* is an abnormal posture in which the patient's arms are adducted and extended, the wrists are pronated, the fingers are flexed, the legs are stiffly extended, and the feet are plantarflexed. **(M-S)**

▷ The best communication tool the nurse can develop is an effective listening technique. **(FND)**

▷ Cerebrospinal fluid is a transcellular fluid. **(M-S)**

▷ Sodium regulates extracellular osmolality. **(M-S)**

▶ In the early stages of shock, the heart and brain maintain blood circulation. **(FND)**

▶ Narcotics may not effectively relieve "phantom" pain. **(M-S)**

▶ The trauma patient who has received multiple blood transfusions is at risk for hypocalcemia and hypothermia. **(M-S)**

▶ In a precipitous labor, delivery is unusually rapid, occurring only 2 hours after labor onset. **(MAT)**

▶ The nurse should advise the woman on oral contraceptives not to smoke. **(M-S)**

▶ Cold constricts blood vessels on the body's surface. **(FND)**

▶ Giving a tepid sponge bath reduces the patient's body temperature. **(FND)**

▶ When applying heat or cold, the nurse should take measures to protect the patient from possible thermal injury. **(FND)**

▶ Moist heat applications heat the skin more quickly than dry heat applications. **(FND)**

▶ For a soak, water temperature shouldn't exceed 105° F (40.5° C). **(FND)**

▶ Infants and geriatric patients have reduced resistance to heat. **(FND)**

▶ After applying an ice pack, the nurse should discontinue the treatment if the patient's skin becomes white or extremely red. **(FND)**

▶ Kernig's sign indicates meningitis. **(M-S)**

▶ A herniated nucleus pulposus (intervertebral disk) most commonly occurs in the lumbar and lumbosacral regions. **(M-S)**

▶ *Laminectomy* is surgical removal of a herniated portion of an intervertebral disk. **(M-S)**

▶ In the patient with a fractured and displaced femur, treatment starts with reduction and immobilization of the affected leg. **(M-S)**

▶ *Flight of ideas* is altered thought processes marked by skipping from one topic to an unrelated topic. **(PSY)**

▶ The patient with conversion disorder may display *la belle indifference*, a lack of concern about an overwhelming disorder, such as blindness or paralysis. **(PSY)**

▶ *Valsalva's maneuver* is forced exhalation against a closed glottis. **(M-S)**

▶ Administering chlorpromazine hydrochloride (Thorazine) to the patient with alcohol intoxication may lead to oversedation and respiratory depression. **(M-S)**

▶ Vital organ perfusion is seriously compromised when mean arterial pressure falls below 60 mm Hg and systolic blood pressure drops below 80 mm Hg. **(M-S)**

▶ Lidocaine hydrochloride (Xylocaine) is the drug of choice for treating premature ventricular contractions. **(M-S)**

▶ The heart's ventricles usually sustain the greatest damage during a myocardial infarction. **(M-S)**

▶ During a myocardial infarction, pain results from myocardial ischemia caused by anoxia. **(M-S)**

▶ The leading cause of death in burn victims is respiratory compromise. **(M-S)**

▶ Prolactin overproduction by the pituitary gland can cause galactorrhea and amenorrhea. **(M-S)**

▶ When using Clark's rule, the nurse multiplies the adult dosage by the child's weight in pounds and then divides the result by 150. **(PED)**

▶ When using Young's rule, the nurse multiplies the adult dosage by the child's age in years and then divides the result by the sum of the child's age plus 12 years. **(PED)**

▶ A *laceration* is a torn, jagged, or irregular wound. **(FND)**

▶ Wristdrop results from paralysis of the extensor muscles in the forearm and hand. **(M-S)**

▶ Footdrop results from excessive plantarflexion; usually, it's a complication of prolonged bed rest. **(M-S)**

▶ In *floating*, the fetal presenting part isn't engaged in the pelvic inlet but is freely movable above the inlet. **(MAT)**

▶ *Engagement* occurs when the largest diameter of the fetal presenting part passes through the pelvic inlet. **(MAT)**

▶ In a Z-track injection, the needle track is sealed off after the injection, minimizing skin irritation and staining. **(FND)**

▶ *Fetal station* indicates the relationship of the fetal presenting part to the maternal ischial spines; the number represents centimeters above or below the spines. **(MAT)**

▶ A presenting part above the ischial spines is designated as fetal station -1, -2, -3, or -4, while a presenting part below the ischial spines is designated as fetal station +1, +2, +3, or +4.   **(MAT)**

▶ At fetal station 0, the largest diameter of the presenting part is level with the ischial spines.   **(MAT)**

▶ The nurse should assess the neonate for the Moro reflex.   **(MAT)**

▶ *Echolalia* is the parrotlike repetition of another person's words or phrases.   **(PSY)**

▶ The *ego* is the rational element of the personality that maintains conscious contact with reality.   **(PSY)**

▶ The *superego* is the partly conscious portion of the psyche that represents internalization of parental conscience and societal rules; it evaluates thoughts and actions, rewarding the good and punishing the bad.   **(PSY)**

▶ The *id* is the unconscious part of the psyche that serves as the source of instinctual energy, impulses, and drives.   **(PSY)**

▶ Ovulation stops during pregnancy.   **(MAT)**

▶ Vaginal bleeding is the most significant danger sign during pregnancy.   **(MAT)**

▶ In the patient who can't void, the nurse should assess the bladder first by palpation.   **(M-S)**

▶ Infants younger than age 1 shouldn't receive cow's milk because of its low linoleic acid and protein content.   **(PED)**

▶ The patient who uses a cane should carry it on the unaffected side.   **(FND)**

▶ *Chloasma,* or *melasma,* is a tan or brownish skin pigmentation that commonly occurs during pregnancy.   **(MAT)**

▶ The nurse should advise pregnant patients that no amount of alcohol intake is safe during pregnancy.   **(MAT)**

▶ Vitamin C deficiency causes brittle bones, pinpoint peripheral hemorrhages, and friable gums with loose teeth.   **(M-S)**

▶ Seclusion is used in psychiatric settings to ensure the patient's safety.   **(PSY)**

▶ Cool, moist, pale skin occurring during shock results from diversion of blood from the skin to major organs.   **(M-S)**

▶ *Validation* is a communication process in which the nurse confirms with the patient that the nurse has understood him. **(FND)**

▶ Fetal alcohol syndrome manifests within the first 24 hours after birth. **(MAT)**

▶ Leukemia is the most common form of cancer in children. **(M-S)**

▶ *Variability* is any change in the fetal heart rate from the normal rate of 120 to 160 beats/minute. **(MAT)**

▶ Hexachlorophene (pHisoHex) is no longer used to bathe infants because it may cause neurotoxicity. **(PED)**

▶ Rapid onset of high fever is a classic first sign of toxic shock syndrome. **(M-S)**

▶ The nurse should provide a dark, quiet environment for the neonate experiencing narcotics withdrawal. **(PED)**

▶ To assess jaundice in the neonate, the nurse should apply slight pressure to cause blanching of the tip of the nose or the gum line and then watch for yellow discoloration after releasing the pressure. **(MAT)**

▶ In the child, the normal fasting blood glucose level is 60 to 100 mg/dl. **(PED)**

▶ If the body can't use glucose for energy production, it metabolizes fat for energy, resulting in ketone production. **(M-S)**

▶ Nostril flaring is the first sign of respiratory distress in the premature neonate. **(MAT)**

▶ The infant's first emotional response is the need for affection. **(PED)**

▶ Having an imaginary friend and speaking to this friend are normal behaviors in 3-year-old children. **(PED)**

▶ The first immunizations the child should receive are hepatitis vaccine, diphtheria and tetanus toxoids and pertussis vaccine, and polio vaccine. **(PED)**

▶ The nurse should assess for electrolyte imbalances in the infant who has had diarrhea six to eight times a day for 4 consecutive days. **(PED)**

▶ Cough medicines containing codeine help to suppress the cough reflex. **(FND)**

▶ Aminophylline and theophylline are bronchodilators. **(M-S)**

▶ Chest percussion helps to loosen bronchial secretions. **(FND)**

▶ Skinfold measurements are used to evaluate the patient's subcutaneous fat stores. **(FND)**

▶ Medulloblastomas typically occur in the cerebellum. **(M-S)**

▶ The patient with diabetic ketoacidosis is at risk for developing shock. **(M-S)**

▶ The patient with diabetes mellitus is susceptible to atherosclerosis. **(M-S)**

▶ Instilling phenylephrine hydrochloride (Neo-Synephrine) into the patient's eye should cause mydriasis. **(M-S)**

▶ When assessing distance vision, the nurse should have the patient stand 20' (6.1 m) from the vision chart. **(FND)**

▶ An elixir, used mainly as a vehicle for an oral drug, contains alcohol, sweeteners, or flavorings. **(M-S)**

▶ The basal metabolic rate is the amount of energy needed to maintain vital body functions. **(M-S)**

▶ Basal metabolic rate is expressed in calories consumed per hour per kilogram of body weight. **(M-S)**

▶ Tetany may result from hypocalcemia. **(M-S)**

▶ Alcohol interferes with the absorption of vitamin B_{12} in the GI tract. **(M-S)**

▶ Proteins are the major sources of building material for muscles, blood, skin, hair, nails, and internal organs. **(FND)**

▶ When taking clomipramine (Anafranil) for depression, the patient should use a sunblock to prevent a photosensitivity reaction. **(M-S)**

▶ Red blood cells transport hemoglobin, white blood cells fight infection, and platelets promote coagulation. **(FND)**

▶ A *compulsion* is an irresistible urge to perform an irrational act, such as walking in a clockwise circle before leaving a room. **(PSY)**

▶ The therapeutic serum level for lithium is 0.6 to 1.2 mEq/L. **(PSY)**

▶ *Habitual abortion* is said to occur when a woman has three or more consecutive spontaneous abortions (also called miscarriages). **(MAT)**

▶ Potassium is the most abundant cation in intracellular fluid. **(M-S)**

▶ A lymph node biopsy revealing Reed-Sternberg cells definitively diagnoses Hodgkin's disease. **(M-S)**

▶ The saliva of the patient with rabies contains the rabies virus and thus poses a hazard for nurses caring for the patient. **(M-S)**

▶ A four-point (quad) cane is indicated for the patient who needs more stability than a regular cane can offer. **(M-S)**

▶ Excessive sedation may cause respiratory depression. **(M-S)**

▶ The intraoperative period starts when the patient is moved to the operating room bed and ends when he's admitted to the postanesthesia recovery unit. **(M-S)**

▶ The nurse's primary postoperative concern is maintaining a patent airway. **(M-S)**

▶ Cyanosis in the circumoral area, sublingual region, or nailbeds signals an oxygen saturation level below 80%. **(M-S)**

▶ During the postoperative period, the nurse should instruct the patient to cough and deep-breathe every 2 hours. **(M-S)**

▶ During the patient's first postoperative ambulation, the nurse should keep a close watch and assist as needed. **(M-S)**

▶ Hypovolemia occurs when 15% to 25% of the body's total blood volume is lost. **(M-S)**

▶ In postoperative patients, the organism most likely to cause septicemia is *Escherichia coli*. **(M-S)**

▶ Teenage mothers are at increased risk for having low birth weight neonates. **(MAT)**

▶ Before drawing blood for arterial blood gas measurement, the nurse should check the patient's collateral blood supply by performing Allen's test. **(M-S)**

▶ A drug has three names: (1) a generic name, (2) a trade, or brand, name, and (3) a chemical name. **(FND)**

▶ The nurse should keep suction equipment at the bedside of the patient who is recovering from maxillofacial surgery. **(M-S)**

▶ *Bestiality* is sexual relations between a human being and an animal. **(PSY)**

▶ *Crowning* is the appearance of the fetus's head as it becomes visible at the vulvovaginal ring and its largest diameter is encircled. **(MAT)**

▶ If an immunization schedule is interrupted for any reason, it should resume from the last immunization administered, not from the beginning. **(PED)**

▶ Exercises that one person performs on another are called *passive*. **(FND)**

▶ Exercises that one person performs against the resistance of another are called *resistive*. **(FND)**

▶ In *isometric* exercises, the person contracts the muscles without moving the affected body part. **(FND)**

▶ Activities of daily living (ADLs) are the activities a person performs during the course of a normal day. **(FND)**

▶ When begun, cardiopulmonary resuscitation shouldn't be interrupted unless the rescuer is alone and must stop to get help. **(M-S)**

▶ The tongue is the most common cause of airway obstruction in unconscious patients. **(M-S)**

▶ For one- and two-rescuer cardiopulmonary resuscitation on an adult, 80 to 100 chest compressions should be delivered per minute. **(M-S)**

▶ In balloon angioplasty, a small, balloon-tipped catheter is inflated inside an artery to exert pressure against a plaque and thus flatten it. **(M-S)**

▶ The patient with a stomach ulcer should avoid bedtime snacks because food may stimulate nocturnal gastric secretions. **(M-S)**

▶ A clear liquid diet consists of clear fluids and foods that become liquid at body temperature. **(FND)**

▶ A full liquid diet, which consists of simple, easily digested foods, is used to provide fluids and calories but may be inadequate in folic acid, iron, vitamin B_6, and fiber. **(FND)**

▶ A pureed diet supplies all of the patient's nutritional needs. **(M-S)**

▶ A *soft diet* includes semisolid foods and is often supplemented with between-meal snacks. **(FND)**

▶ A *mechanical soft diet* is used for the patient who has difficulty chewing or tolerating a regular diet. **(FND)**

▶ The patient who requires no dietary modifications can receive a regular diet. **(FND)**

▶ The doctor normally orders a "diet for age" for the pediatric patient. **(PED)**

▶ A bland diet doesn't include foods that cause gastric irritation or excess acid secretions unless these provide a neutralizing effect. **(FND)**

▶ The patient with a gastric ulcer should avoid alcohol, caffeinated beverages, aspirin, and spicy foods. **(M-S)**

▶ Bacteria that convert penicillin into an inactive product produce the enzyme penicillinase. **(M-S)**

▶ Staphylococcal or streptococcal organisms cause impetigo contagiosa. **(M-S)**

▶ *Battle's sign* is a bluish discoloration or bruising over the mastoid area. **(M-S)**

▶ Antibiotics are ineffective against viruses, protozoa, and parasites. **(M-S)**

▶ Natural penicillins inhibit synthesis of the bacterial cell wall. **(M-S)**

▶ Aminoglycosides are natural antibiotics that are effective against gram-negative bacteria. **(M-S)**

▶ When caring for the patient receiving aminoglycosides, the nurse should watch for nephrotoxicity and ototoxicity. **(M-S)**

▶ In phimosis, the foreskin can't be retracted over the glans penis. **(PED)**

▶ The patient with a strangulated hernia typically complains of pain, nausea, and vomiting. **(M-S)**

▶ In chronic prostatitis, the prostate gland is enlarged, tender, and somewhat boggy. **(M-S)**

▶ The heart of the child with tetralogy of Fallot appears boot-shaped on X-ray because of the enlarged right ventricle. **(PED)**

▶ The six cardinal positions of gaze evaluate the function of all extraocular muscles and cranial nerves III, IV, and VI. **(M-S)**

▶ A *hordeolum* (stye) is an inflammation of the eyelid margin originating in a sebaceous gland of an eyelash. **(M-S)**

▶ A *chalazion* is a chronic eyelid inflammation caused by an obstructed meibomian gland. **(M-S)**

▶ Respiratory acidosis may occur in such conditions as drug overdose, Guillain-Barré syndrome, myasthenia gravis, and chronic obstructive pulmonary disease. **(M-S)**

▶ Respiratory alkalosis may occur in such conditions as high fever, severe hypoxia, asthma, and pulmonary embolism. **(M-S)**

▶ Metabolic acidosis may result from renal failure, diarrhea, diabetic ketosis, and lactic ketosis. **(M-S)**

▶ Metabolic alkalosis may result from nasal and gastric suctioning, excessive diuretic use, and steroid therapy. **(M-S)**

▶ Heart murmurs occur in six grades, designated I through VI. **(M-S)**

▶ The nurse can hear a grade VI heart murmur with the stethoscope raised slightly above the patient's chest. **(M-S)**

▶ The "six Fs" of abdominal distention are *flatus, feces, fetus, fluid, fat,* and *fatal growth neoplasm.* **(FND)**

▶ Murphy's sign indicates acute cholecystitis. **(M-S)**

▶ Psoas sign (abdominal rigidity and rebound tenderness) indicates appendicitis. **(M-S)**

▶ The nurse can detect ascites by checking for a fluid wave in the abdomen or by percussing the abdomen for shifting dullness. **(FND)**

▶ The patient's goal is the most important goal to incorporate into the nursing plan of care. **(FND)**

▶ A stable environment helps minimize confusion in the patient with organic brain syndrome. **(PSY)**

▶ Typically, the patient with organic brain syndrome loses recent memory first. **(PSY)**

▶ The Apgar score evaluates the neonate's respiratory effort, heart rate, muscle tone, reflex irritability, and color. **(MAT)**

▶ During cardiac catheterization, the patient may experience a thudding sensation in the chest from catheter manipulation. **(M-S)**

▶ During the third trimester of pregnancy, the anti-insulin effects of placental hormones increase the patient's insulin needs. **(MAT)**

▶ The biparietal diameter of the fetal head is used to assess gestational age during ultrasound. **(MAT)**

▶ Congenital malformations are common in neonates of diabetic mothers. **(MAT)**

▶ Nutritional deficiency is a common finding in patients with a long-standing history of alcohol abuse. **(PSY)**

▶ The alcoholic patient typically receives thiamine to slow the progression of peripheral neuropathy. **(PSY)**

▶ The patient experiencing alcohol withdrawal may receive sedatives to prevent delirium tremens. **(PSY)**

▶ Alcohol lowers the seizure threshold in certain people. **(PSY)**

▶ *Paraphrasing* is an active listening technique in which the nurse restates the message the patient has just conveyed. **(FND)**

▶ During the *preicteric phase* of hepatitis A, early signs and symptoms include headache, malaise, fatigue, lassitude, anorexia, and fever. **(M-S)**

▶ Most patients with hepatitis A are asymptomatic. **(M-S)**

▶ Hepatitis A usually spreads by the fecal-oral route. **(M-S)**

▶ A significant rise in serum transaminase is characteristic in both hepatitis A and hepatitis B. **(M-S)**

▶ Excessive vomiting or removal of stomach contents through suctioning can reduce body potassium stores, leading to hypokalemia. **(M-S)**

▶ During a follow-up examination of the patient who is a purified-protein-derivative converter, the nurse should determine if the patient has experienced any signs or symptoms of tuberculosis. **(M-S)**

▶ Signs of acute rheumatic fever include chorea, fever, carditis, migratory polyarthritis, skin rash, and subcutaneous nodules. **(M-S)**

▶ The patient with a history of rheumatic fever should take prophylactic antibiotics before undergoing dental work or other invasive procedures. **(M-S)**

▶ The patient on a low-residue diet should avoid fruits because they are high in fiber and low in protein. **(M-S)**

▶ Postoperative pain peaks during the first 24 hours after surgery. **(M-S)**

▶ After a myocardial infarction, most patients are permitted to resume sexual activity when they can climb two flights of stairs without fatigue or dyspnea. **(M-S)**

▶ Geriatric patients are more prone to orthostatic hypotension than younger patients. **(M-S)**

▶ Buttocks tightening is a perineal exercise that strengthens the pelvic muscles. **(M-S)**

▶ When two psychiatric patients are engaged in escalating hostilities, the nurse should diffuse the situation by sending both patients to their rooms and providing one-on-one therapy. **(PSY)**

▶ Many preterm neonates have immature swallowing and sucking reflexes. **(MAT)**

▶ The nurse should strain the urine of the patient with suspected renal or urethral calculi to determine if any stones have passed. **(M-S)**

▶ The nurse should inventory and safeguard the personal belongings of the deceased adult patient. **(FND)**

▶ To maximize lung expansion, the nurse should place the patient with ascites in semi-Fowler's position. **(M-S)**

▶ When caring for the patient who has ingested poison, the nurse should save any vomitus for analysis. **(M-S)**

▶ Acrocyanosis and cool extremities are normal findings in neonates. **(MAT)**

▶ The earliest signs of respiratory distress are restlessness and an increased respiratory rate, followed by an increased heart rate. **(M-S)**

▶ Vomiting within 4 hours after a meal may result from food intoxication (from bacterial toxins). **(M-S)**

▶ Vomiting, fever, and diarrhea arising 12 to 18 hours after a meal suggest food poisoning. **(M-S)**

▶ Acute meningitis causes elevated levels of protein in cerebrospinal fluid. **(M-S)**

▶ The patient receiving loop diuretics should supplement his diet with foods containing potassium. **(M-S)**

▶ With the confused patient, maintaining consistency in nursing staff is paramount. **(PSY)**

▶ *Hypercapnia* refers to an excess of carbon dioxide in the blood. **(M-S)**

▶ Vasopressin and oxytocin are secreted by the posterior pituitary gland. **(M-S)**

▶ The three meninges are the dura mater, pia mater, and arachnoid. **(M-S)**

▶ Milk shouldn't be included in a clear liquid diet. **(FND)**

▶ Tetracycline, silver nitrate, or erythromycin should be instilled in a neonate's eyes to prevent gonorrhea. **(MAT)**

▶ When using crutches, the patient should bear weight on the hands. **(FND)**

▶ The female reproductive organs normally affected by gonorrhea are the vagina and fallopian tubes. **(M-S)**

▶ After surgery to correct a retinal detachment, the patient should avoid sudden movement, such as sneezing or bending over. **(M-S)**

▶ Hemorrhage is the most common postoperative problem. **(M-S)**

▶ Kussmaul's respirations represent the body's attempt to "blow off" excess carbon dioxide. **(M-S)**

▶ Phenylketonuria is an inborn error of metabolism of phenylalanine. **(PED)**

▶ Epinephrine hydrochloride is a sympathomimetic drug that acts primary on $alpha_1$, $beta_1$, and $beta_2$ receptors. **(M-S)**

▶ Adverse effects of epinephrine hydrochloride include tachycardia, palpitations, headache, and hypertension. **(M-S)**

▶ Psychologists, physical therapists, and chiropractors aren't authorized to write prescriptions. **(FND)**

▶ The nurse should use mild soap and water to clean the skin around a stoma. **(M-S)**

▶ Green, leafy vegetables are high in fiber. **(FND)**

▶ A cardinal sign of acute pancreatitis is an elevated serum amylase level. **(M-S)**

▶ During a colostomy irrigation, painful cramps may result from a rapid flow rate. **(M-S)**

▶ The patient can control some of the odor associated with a colostomy by avoiding such foods as fish, eggs, onions, beans, and cabbage. **(M-S)**

▶ The average child requires a 25G to 27G ½" needle for subcutaneous injections. **(PED)**

▶ When giving a subcutaneous injection of less than 1 ml of a drug, the nurse should always use a tuberculin syringe. **(FND)**

▶ The nurse must identify the patient by checking his identification band before administering any medication. **(FND)**

▶ Before giving an injection, the nurse should clean the skin at the injection site with a sterile alcohol sponge, starting at the center and moving outward in circles. **(FND)**

▶ If blood is aspirated into the syringe before an I.M. injection, the nurse should withdraw the needle and prepare another syringe. **(FND)**

▶ After an injection, the nurse should apply pressure to stop any bleeding from the injection site. **(FND)**

▶ The nurse should never tweeze the patient's eyebrows or dye the patient's hair. **(FND)**

▶ When providing hair and scalp care, the nurse should start combing at the ends of the hair and work toward the scalp. **(FND)**

▶ The nurse shouldn't cut the patient's hair without written consent from the patient, parent, or guardian. **(FND)**

▶ When washing the hands, the nurse need not remove a wedding ring but should remove a watch and other jewelry. **(FND)**

▶ When caring for a hearing-impaired patient, the nurse should raise the voice moderately but shouldn't shout. **(FND)**

▶ Redness after heat lamp application indicates a skin burn. **(M-S)**

▶ The nurse should remove the patient's heel protectors every 8 hours to expose the heels to air and assess the skin. **(M-S)**

▶ Hot soaks promote drainage and relieve pain from inflammation. **(FND)**

▶ The most common sexually transmitted disease in the United States is *Chlamydia*. **(M-S)**

▶ In the female patient, signs of chlamydial infection include a positive culture, urinary frequency, greenish white vaginal discharge, and cervical inflammation. **(M-S)**

▶ The pituitary gland is located in the sella turcica of the sphenoid bone in the cranial cavity. **(M-S)**

▶ Healing by secondary intention occurs with large wounds that cause significant tissue loss. **(M-S)**

▶ In healing by first intention, union or continuity occurs directly; wound edges are well approximated, usually with sutures. **(M-S)**

▶ Myasthenia gravis typically affects young females. **(M-S)**

▶ Patients with anorexia nervosa must be observed during meals and for several hours afterward. **(PSY)**

▶ The child with untreated phenylketonuria fails to reach early developmental milestones. **(PED)**

▶ Degenerative joint disease is the most common form of arthritis that affects almost all joints. **(M-S)**

▶ Progressive deterioration and loss of articular cartilage characterize osteoarthritis. **(M-S)**

▶ Reactive arthritis typically causes conjunctivitis and urethritis as well as arthritis. **(M-S)**

▶ Foods high in carbohydrates are quickly digested, more readily emptied from the stomach into the duodenum, and more likely to cause diarrhea. **(M-S)**

▶ Immediately following delivery, the nurse should suction the neonate's nose after suctioning the mouth. **(MAT)**

▶ Drying the neonate immediately after delivery helps maintain body heat by preventing heat loss through evaporation. **(MAT)**

▶ When bathing the infant, the nurse should expose only one body part at a time. **(MAT)**

▶ To promote bonding, the patient should be permitted to breast-feed her neonate on the delivery table if she desires. **(MAT)**

▶ The nurse should measure the neonate's temperature at least every 2 hours. **(MAT)**

▶ Typically, the neonate weighs 5½ to 9 lb and measures 18″ to 22″ long. **(MAT)**

▶ To test nares patency, the nurse should try to elicit a sneeze from the neonate. **(MAT)**

▶ *Epstein's pearls* (also called pseudodiphtheria) are small, whitish yellow lesions that may appear on either side of the neonate's throat; they're considered normal and disappear without treatment. **(MAT)**

▶ Supernumerary nipples occasionally appear on neonates and may be mistaken for moles. **(MAT)**

▶ The neonate's spine should be straight. **(MAT)**

▶ *Polydactyly* refers to extra fingers or toes. **(M-S)**

▶ Babinski's reflex is normal in the neonate and may persist for up to 18 months. **(MAT)**

▶ In the *extrusion reflex,* the infant spits out food placed on the front of the tongue. **(PED)**

▶ *Harlequin sign* is reddening of the lower half of the body and pallor of the upper half in the neonate lying on his side. **(MAT)**

▶ *Mongolian spots* are blue-black macules seen on the sacrum and buttocks of some neonates. **(MAT)**

▶ *Vernix caseosa* is a cheeselike substance that covers the skin of the neonate. **(MAT)**

▶ A *fugue state* is an extreme form of amnesia accompanied by flight from familiar surroundings; the person may take on a new identity. **(PSY)**

▶ *Caput succedaneum* in the fetus is scalp swelling that may overlie the sutures of the skull, usually occurring during labor from pressure exerted by the cervix. **(MAT)**

▶ *Nevus flammeus* (also called port-wine stain) is a diffuse lesion ranging from pink to dark bluish red that may appear on the neonate's face or thighs. **(MAT)**

▶ *Strawberry hemangiomas* are raised, red birthmarks that generally disappear by age 1. **(MAT)**

▶ *Cavernous hemangiomas* resemble strawberry hemangiomas but don't disappear with age. **(M-S)**

▶ When administering penicillin G procaine I.M. to the adult, the nurse should inject the needle deep into the upper outer quadrant of the buttock. **(M-S)**

▶ For the neonate's first bottle-feeding, the nurse should give a few sips of sterile water, followed by 1 oz of glucose water. **(MAT)**

▶ To help establish the mother's milk supply pattern, the breast-fed neonate should be fed at least every 2 to 3 hours. **(MAT)**

▶ The nurse should wear gloves when giving the neonate his first bath. **(MAT)**

▶ The neonate with a suspected infection should be isolated. **(PED)**

▶ The Schilling test confirms pernicious anemia. **(M-S)**

▶ A colostomy in the ascending colon drains fluid fecal matter. **(M-S)**

▶ A colostomy in the descending colon drains solid fecal matter.
(M-S)

▶ The patient undergoing chemotherapy should eat a diet high in calories and protein. **(M-S)**

▶ Chemotherapy may cause hair loss. **(M-S)**

▶ The infant with celiac disease has fatty, foul-smelling stools. **(PED)**

▶ The results of hemoglobin electrophoresis differentiate sickle cell trait from sickle cell anemia. **(M-S)**

▶ The Sickledex, or sickle cell prep, is a diagnostic test used only to detect sickle cells in blood. **(M-S)**

▶ *Eruption* refers to a tooth breaking out from the dental crypt through surrounding tissue. **(PED)**

▶ A folded towel (scrotal bridge) can be used to provide scrotal support.
(M-S)

▶ Supine hypotension syndrome in the pregnant patient results from pressure exerted by the enlarging uterus, which decreases venous return. **(MAT)**

▶ The nurse should advise the pregnant patient with ankle edema to take frequent rests, elevate the feet, and avoid constrictive clothing.
(MAT)

▶ When the doctor orders "diet as tolerated," the nurse should progress the patient's diet as follows: (1) clear liquids, (2) full liquids, (3) soft diet, and (4) regular (house) diet. **(M-S)**

▶ Drinking too much plain water can lead to electrolyte imbalances.
(FND)

▶ The patient has the right to accept or refuse treatment. **(FND)**

▶ Illness or injury may cause a person to regress to a lower level of functioning. **(FND)**

▶ Health is a state of physiologic and psychological well-being. **(FND)**

▶ In naturally acquired active immunity, antibodies are produced on exposure to a microorganism. **(M-S)**

▶ Naturally acquired passive immunity occurs when the fetus receives antibodies from the mother. **(MAT)**

▶ In artificially acquired immunity, the person is infected with weakened or dead microorganisms or an inactive form of the organism's toxin. **(M-S)**

▶ The major tissue types are epithelial, connective, muscle, and nerve tissue. **(M-S)**

▶ Cells are the body's basic structural unit. **(FND)**

▶ During the aging process, bones lose calcium and become brittle; this, in turn, increases the risk for fractures and poor healing after a fracture. **(FND)**

▶ Because dermal skin damage causes loss of the skin's mitotic structures, the damaged dermis takes longer to heal than the damaged epidermis. **(M-S)**

▶ Diffusion, osmosis, and filtration are passive transport processes. **(M-S)**

▶ The main types of muscle tissue are skeletal (voluntary), smooth (involuntary), and cardiac muscle tissue. **(M-S)**

▶ Neurons respond to stimuli and transmit nerve impulses. **(M-S)**

▶ Neuroglia support and connect nervous tissue but don't transmit nerve impulses. **(M-S)**

▶ Multiple sclerosis causes deterioration of the myelin sheath of the central nervous system. **(M-S)**

▶ The body has 31 pairs of spinal nerves. **(M-S)**

▶ The thyroid gland controls the rate of metabolism. **(M-S)**

▶ The parathyroid gland regulates serum calcium and phosphorus levels. **(M-S)**

▶ Blood is composed of plasma and formed elements (white blood cells, red blood cells, and platelets). **(M-S)**

▶ The patient who has been on "nothing by mouth" status for 3 or more days without receiving nutritional support is at risk for nutritional deficits. **(M-S)**

▶ If the patient complains of nausea or starts to choke or vomit during a tube feeding, the nurse should stop the feeding immediately and call the doctor. **(M-S)**

▶ The nurse should check the patient's distal pulses before and after splinting a fracture. **(M-S)**

▶ Rescuers performing cardiopulmonary resuscitation on a child should deliver 100 chest compressions per minute. **(PED)**

▶ The patient with a completely obstructed airway can't talk, breathe, or cough. **(M-S)**

▶ The courts are likely to assume that nursing care that wasn't documented wasn't given. **(FND)**

▶ During skin testing, the nurse should keep epinephrine and emergency equipment available. **(M-S)**

▶ Alcohol is a central nervous system depressant. **(M-S)**

▶ Gangrene usually affects the fingers and toes first. **(M-S)**

▶ In the infant, a sunken fontanel is one of the first signs of dehydration. **(PED)**

▶ The trauma victim shouldn't be moved until a patent airway has been established and the cervical spine has been immobilized. **(M-S)**

▶ Rescuers should place the victim on a solid, flat surface before administering cardiopulmonary resuscitation. **(M-S)**

▶ Brain damage occurs 4 to 6 minutes after cardiopulmonary function ceases. **(M-S)**

▶ An adrenalectomy may decrease steroid production, which in turn may lead to extensive sodium and water loss. **(M-S)**

▶ In the healthy person, fluid intake should roughly equal fluid losses. **(M-S)**

▶ The body's major buffer system is the bicarbonate buffer. **(M-S)**

▶ Metabolic acidosis results from excessive loss of bicarbonate or excessive production or retention of acid. **(M-S)**

▶ *Hemianopsia* is blindness or defective vision in half the visual field of one or both eyes. **(FND)**

▶ After a fracture of the epiphyseal plate, the child may suffer growth disturbances, such as bone shortening or overgrowth. **(PED)**

▶ An acetaminophen overdose can severely damage the liver. **(M-S)**

▶ Prominent signs of advanced cirrhosis are ascites and jaundice. **(M-S)**

▶ *Somnambulism* is sleepwalking. **(M-S)**

▶ Epinephrine is a vasoconstrictor. **(M-S)**

▶ Stress management is a short-term goal of psychotherapy.   **(PSY)**

▶ Penicillin should be administered 1 to 2 hours before or 2 to 3 hours after a meal.   **(M-S)**

▶ To ensure accurate central venous pressure readings, the nurse should place the manometer or transducer level with the phlebostatic axis.   **(M-S)**

▶ Arterial blood is bright red, flows rapidly, and spurts with each heartbeat because it's pumped directly from the heart.   **(M-S)**

▶ Venous blood is dark red and tends to ooze from a wound.   **(M-S)**

▶ Signs and symptoms of anaphylaxis commonly stem from histamine release.   **(M-S)**

▶ Urine pH above 8.0 can result from a urinary tract infection, a highly alkaline diet, or systemic alkalosis.   **(M-S)**

▶ Urine pH below 4.5 may indicate a high-protein diet, fever, or metabolic acidosis.   **(M-S)**

▶ Signs of accessory muscle use include shoulder elevation, intercostal muscle retraction, and scalene and sternocleidomastoid muscle use during respiration.   **(M-S)**

▶ *Lanugo* covering the fetus's body is almost entirely shed by the 9th month.   **(MAT)**

▶ If wound dehiscence occurs, the nurse should cover the wound with a moist, sterile dressing and notify the doctor.   **(M-S)**

▶ A rash is the most common allergic reaction to penicillin.   **(M-S)**

▶ Atropine sulfate blocks the effects of acetylcholine.   **(M-S)**

▶ Patent ductus arteriosus is an acyanotic congenital heart defect.   **(M-S)**

▶ Salicylates are the drugs of choice for treating rheumatoid arthritis.   **(M-S)**

▶ Deep, intense pain that usually worsens at night and is unrelated to movement suggests bone pain.   **(M-S)**

▶ Pain that follows prolonged or excessive exercise and subsides with rest suggests muscle pain.   **(M-S)**

▶ Mannitol (Osmitrol) is an osmotic diuretic.   **(M-S)**

▶ The biophysical profile is a scoring system used to assess fetal well-being.   **(MAT)**

▶ The five activities of the digestive system are ingestion, food propulsion, digestion, absorption, and elimination. **(FND)**

▶ TORCH infections include *t*oxoplasmosis, *o*ther infections (chlamydia, group B beta-hemolytic streptococcus, syphilis, and varicella zoster), *r*ubella, *c*ytomegalovirus, and *h*erpesviruses. **(M-S)**

▶ Before transferring the patient from a bed to a wheelchair, the nurse should push the wheelchair's footrests to the sides and lock the wheels. **(FND)**

▶ The tetralogy of Fallot consists of four defects: (1) ventricular septal defect, (2) overriding aorta, (3) pulmonic stenosis, and (4) right ventricular hypertrophy. **(PED)**

▶ Red cell indices aid in diagnosing anemias. **(M-S)**

▶ An exercise stress test continues until the patient reaches a predetermined target heart rate or experiences chest pain, fatigue, or other signs or symptoms of exercise intolerance. **(M-S)**

▶ The therapeutic blood level for digoxin is 0.5 to 2.5 ng/ml. **(M-S)**

▶ Under the Controlled Substances Act, the pharmacy must account for every dose of a controlled drug it dispenses. **(FND)**

▶ Jaundice is a sign of dysfunction, not a disease in itself. **(M-S)**

▶ Most patients with type 2 diabetes mellitus don't need exogenous insulin. **(M-S)**

▶ Intermediate-acting insulins peak in 4 to 15 hours. **(M-S)**

▶ Long-acting insulins peak in 10 to 30 hours. **(M-S)**

▶ Hypoglycemia occurs when the blood glucose level falls below 50 mg/dl. **(M-S)**

▶ Hypoglycemia may occur 1 to 3 hours after administration of a rapid-acting insulin. **(M-S)**

▶ A rapid drop in the blood glucose level may cause sweating, tremors, pallor, and tachycardia. **(M-S)**

▶ The patient with diabetes mellitus should inspect the feet daily. **(M-S)**

▶ Corrective lenses for nearsightedness are concave. **(M-S)**

▶ Corrective lenses for farsightedness are convex. **(M-S)**

▶ *Refraction* refers to clinical measurement of the refractive errors of the eye. **(FND)**

▶ Adhesions (bands of granulation and scar tissue) develop in some patients after a surgical incision.   **(M-S)**

▶ The nurse should moisten an eye patch when applying it on the unconscious patient.   **(FND)**

▶ The fluorescent treponemal antibody absorption test is a specific serologic test for syphilis.   **(M-S)**

▶ Signs of circulatory interference include abnormally cool skin, cyanosis, and rubor or pallor.   **(M-S)**

▶ The Hoyer lift allows two people to lift and move the nonambulatory patient safely.   **(FND)**

▶ The nurse should use a vest restraint cautiously in the patient with heart failure because it may tighten with movement, further limiting respiratory function.   **(FND)**

▶ The Centers for Disease Control and Prevention recommends using a needleless system when piggybacking an I.V. medication into the main I.V. line.   **(M-S)**

▶ A mask should cover the wearer's mouth and nose; it shouldn't be reused after removal.   **(FND)**

▶ If a gown is required, the nurse should don it before entering the patient's room and discard it on leaving.   **(FND)**

▶ The average duration of pregnancy is 280 days, 40 weeks, 9 calendar months, or 10 lunar months.   **(MAT)**

▶ The nurse should suspect respiratory alkalosis in the patient whose partial pressure of carbon dioxide falls below 35 mm Hg.   **(M-S)**

▶ A *vitamin* is an organic compound that is essential to metabolic processes and can't be synthesized by the body.   **(M-S)**

▶ Peer group is a major influence on the adolescent's eating habits.   **(PED)**

▶ Respiratory tract infections may trigger asthma attacks.   **(M-S)**

▶ Oxygen therapy may be used to prevent or treat hypoxemia in the patient with severe asthma.   **(M-S)**

▶ During an asthma attack, the patient may prefer nasal prongs to a Venturi mask because the mask may have a smothering effect.   **(M-S)**

▶ Cellulitis causes localized heat, redness, swelling, and occasionally, fever, chills, and malaise.   **(M-S)**

▶ The neonate's hemoglobin value normally ranges from 14 to 27 g/dl.
(MAT)

▶ Venous stasis may trigger thrombophlebitis.
(M-S)

▶ *Vitiligo* is a skin disease resulting from pigment cell destruction; it causes irregular skin patches that lack pigment.
(M-S)

▶ Ascites may be detected when more than 500 ml of fluid has accumulated in the intraperitoneal space.
(M-S)

▶ In adults, gastroenteritis is usually self-limiting and causes diarrhea, abdominal discomfort, nausea, and vomiting.
(M-S)

▶ The patient recovering from surgery to correct retinal detachment should avoid sudden movements because they put stress on the suture line.
(M-S)

▶ Taut, shiny skin and edema are signs of fluid volume excess. **(M-S)**

▶ When the patient has suspected food poisoning, the nurse should notify public health authorities, who will take samples of suspected contaminated food and interview the patient, others who ate at the same place, and food handlers.
(M-S)

▶ Down syndrome (trisomy 21) is the most common chromosomal disorder.
(PED)

▶ When determining which information to give the hospitalized child about a procedure, the nurse should consider the child's developmental age.
(PED)

▶ Angiotensin-converting enzyme inhibitors decrease blood pressure by interfering with the renin-angiotensin-aldosterone system. **(M-S)**

▶ An *anion* is an ion that carries a negative electrical charge. **(M-S)**

▶ *Urinary incontinence* refers to the inability to voluntarily control urination.
(M-S)

▶ Patients with spinal cord injury at or above T7 are at risk for autonomic dysreflexia.
(M-S)

▶ *Bradypnea* refers to an abnormally slow rate of breathing. **(FND)**

▶ *Residual volume* refers to the amount of air remaining in the lungs after the deepest possible expiration.
(FND)

▶ Nitrofurantoin (Macrodantin) may turn the urine brown or darker in color.
(M-S)

▶ In a dark-skinned patient, jaundice may not be observable in the sclera. **(FND)**

▶ Handling a wet cast with the fingertips can cause indentations leading to pressure sores. **(FND)**

▶ Informed consent is required for any invasive procedure. **(FND)**

▶ A phenytoin level of 10 to 20 µg/ml is therapeutic. **(M-S)**

▶ In the infant, a key sign of increasing intracranial pressure is bulging fontanels. **(PED)**

▶ On percussion, dullness would be heard over the liver. **(FND)**

▶ In *phantom sensation,* the patient feels as though the missing body part, such as a breast or limb, were still present. **(M-S)**

▶ *Dysfunctional grief* refers to grief that is abnormal or distorted and may be inhibited or unresolved. **(PSY)**

▶ The normal value for arterial blood oxygen saturation is 94% to 100%. **(M-S)**

▶ One milliliter is equivalent to 30 cm³. **(FND)**

▶ When using crutches, bearing weight on the axillae can cause damage to the nerves and circulation in that area. **(FND)**

▶ The Rh-negative woman who isn't sensitized should receive $Rh_o(D)$ immune globulin after an abortion. **(MAT)**

▶ If the patient is receiving propranolol hydrochloride (Inderal), the nurse should tell the patient not to discontinue the drug suddenly because this could exacerbate angina. **(M-S)**

▶ The radial artery is most commonly used to obtain an arterial blood gas. **(M-S)**

▶ The nurse should warn the patient receiving phenytoin (Dilantin) that it may turn the urine pink, red, or reddish brown. **(M-S)**

▶ Feeding patterns for the bottle-fed infant are every 3 to 4 hours on demand. **(PED)**

▶ Measures to prevent transmission of infection include hand washing, barrier precautions, and isolation precautions. **(FND)**

▶ A *syrup* is a drug combined with water and a sugar solution. **(FND)**

▶ The enzyme-linked immunosorbent assay determines the presence of human immunodeficiency virus antibodies and documents exposure to the virus. **(M-S)**

▶ The fourth stage of labor ends with maternal stabilization and lasts 1 to 2 hours. **(MAT)**

▶ Almost all external bleeding can be stopped by direct pressure. **(M-S)**

▶ Verapamil hydrochloride is a calcium channel blocker. **(M-S)**

▶ The postoperative patient who is positioned upright too quickly may complain of light-headedness, dizziness, and fainting. **(M-S)**

▶ *Raynaud's phenomenon* occurs more frequently in colder climates and during the winter months. **(M-S)**

▶ Manifestations of a disulfiram (Antabuse) reaction include flushing, throbbing headache, dyspnea, nausea, vomiting, diaphoresis, chest pain, hyperventilation, hypotension, syncope, weakness, blurred vision, and confusion. **(M-S)**

▶ A consent can be deemed legally insufficient if it can be proven that the patient didn't understand all the facts about a procedure. **(M-S)**

▶ Intact skin and mucous membranes are the body's first line of defense against microorganisms. **(FND)**

▶ The Western blot test identifies the presence of human immunodeficiency virus antibodies and confirms seropositivity of the enzyme-linked immunosorbent assay. **(M-S)**

▶ *Desensitization therapy* gradually exposes the patient to anxiety-provoking or emotionally distressing stimuli. **(PSY)**

▶ One gram of carbohydrate provides 4 calories. **(M-S)**

▶ Because a clear liquid diet is deficient in certain nutrients, it's suitable for only brief periods, typically 24 to 36 hours postoperatively. **(FND)**

▶ When administering heparin subcutaneously, the nurse shouldn't aspirate after injection into the skin. **(M-S)**

▶ The normal serum creatinine level is 0 to 200 mg/24 hours. **(M-S)**

▶ If the patient's feet have gangrene, use a bed cradle to prevent further tissue breakdown. **(FND)**

▶ A low-fat, low-sodium diet could include cold chicken and fresh salad. **(FND)**

▶ A rapid, weak pulse is considered to be thready. **(FND)**

▶ If the patient hasn't signed an informed consent for a procedure, he shouldn't be transferred off the unit to the operating room and the charge nurse should be notified. **(FND)**

▶ Iron medication should be administered after meals. **(FND)**

▶ Atropine sulfate is administered preoperatively to dry up secretions. **(M-S)**

▶ Before a blood transfusion, the patient is routinely given diphenhydramine hydrochloride to minimize transfusion reactions. **(M-S)**

▶ The patient with oral candidiasis should be instructed to keep nystatin (Mycostatin) oral solution in the mouth as long as possible to facilitate contact of the medication with the organism. **(M-S)**

▶ Predisposing factors for oral cancer include smoking cigarettes, chewing tobacco, and drinking alcohol. **(M-S)**

▶ The nurse should inspect the emesis of the patient with an oral cesium or radium radioactive implant to ensure that it wasn't displaced during vomiting. **(M-S)**

▶ *Ecchymosis* means bruised tissue. **(M-S)**

▶ *Erythema* means reddened tissue. **(M-S)**

▶ To minimize and relieve edema, elevate the patient's affected limb and apply ice for 20 minutes on, followed by 20 minutes off. **(M-S)**

▶ When wrapping the ankle with a roller bandage, start at the metatarsals and wrap from the distal to the proximal aspect of the foot. **(FND)**

▶ A consistent finding in the patient with varicose veins is a complaint of achiness, heaviness, and pain in the affected lower extremity. **(M-S)**

▶ Pain on ambulation is called *claudication* and is most likely caused by inadequate arterial blood flow. **(M-S)**

▶ The best method for relieving the pain associated with varicose veins is to elevate the affected lower extremity periodically throughout the day. **(M-S)**

▶ Stasis ulcers first appear as darkly pigmented, scaly areas and progress to skin breakdown and craters that are difficult to heal. **(M-S)**

▶ For the patient who has had vein stripping and vein ligation surgery, the doctor will order walking hourly in the immediate postoperative period. **(M-S)**

▶ Caffeine can impair blood flow because it constricts arteries and arterioles and should be avoided by patients with a history of venous stasis. **(M-S)**

▶ Signs of adequate circulation in an extremity include warm-to-touch toes and feet and capillary refill of less than 3 seconds. **(FND)**

▶ A throat culture is obtained from the posterior pharynx and should be taken while not touching the tongue and mouth with the swab. **(FND)**

▶ The person taking antihistamines should be advised not to drive or use machinery; the medication can make him drowsy and sleepy. **(M-S)**

▶ Clinical manifestations of an anaphylactic reaction include dyspnea, hypotension, hives, and loss of consciousness. **(M-S)**

▶ The treatment for anaphylaxis is epinepherine. **(M-S)**

▶ Sequelae of untreated beta-hemolytic streptococcal infections such as strep throat are glomerulonephritis, rheumatic fever, and rheumatic heart disease. **(M-S)**

▶ The patient with laryngitis should be instructed to rest the larynx by not whispering or talking. **(M-S)**

▶ Parents should be instructed to use cool-mist humidifiers rather than steam to reduce the risk of a scalding injury to the child. **(M-S)**

▶ To minimize the risk of diversional activity deficit in the patient, encourage visits from family and friends and allow the patient to engage in enjoyable activity that is consistent with the treatment plan. **(FND)**

▶ Instruct the patient with an esophageal stricture to chew his food thoroughly; well-chewed food will pass more easily into the stomach. **(M-S)**

▶ The most common symptoms associated with hemolytic blood transfusion reactions are dyspnea, low back pain, constriction in the chest, and hypotension. **(M-S)**

▶ Ineffective infant feeding pattern is the appropriate nursing diagnosis for the infant who can't coordinate sucking, swallowing, and breathing. **(M-S)**

▶ The patient with a hiatal hernia should be instructed to sit upright for at least 2 hours after meals, sleep with his head elevated, and eat small, frequent meals to avoid overextending his stomach. **(M-S)**

▶ The best indication that a patient is being successfully fed by hyperalimentation or gastric feeding is maintenance of prehospital weight or regaining of lost weight. **(M-S)**

▶ Flank pain is a common manifestation of acute pyelonephritis.
(M-S)

▶ Following a gastrostomy, the nurse should expect some serosanguineous draining from the gastrostomy tube. **(M-S)**

▶ Body image disturbance is an appropriate nursing diagnosis for a patient with bronze-like pigmentation on the face secondary to Addison's disease. **(FND)**

▶ Aspirin should be taken with food or milk to prevent gastric irritation. **(M-S)**

▶ Good sources of iron include legumes, liver, leafy green vegetables, dried fruit, and fortified cereals. **(M-S)**

▶ During peritoneal dialysis, the nurse should observe the patient for abdominal distention. **(M-S)**

▶ *Lanugo* is the fine downy hair that often presents on the body of the patient with anorexia nervosa because of a loss of subcutaneous fat. **(MAT)**

▶ Extracorporeal shock wave lithotripsy is a method of pulverizing gallstones with shock waves. **(M-S)**

▶ The patient with undiagnosed abdominal pain shouldn't be given anything by mouth. **(M-S)**

▶ The best method for preventing postoperative respiratory complications is ambulating the patient. **(M-S)**

▶ An increased anodal opening sound is a sign of rheumatic heart disease and rheumatic fever. **(M-S)**

▶ Aspirin is an appropriate drug for the child with rheumatic fever, but it should be withheld and the physician notified if the patient develops a viral infection. **(PED)**

▶ A sign of diabetic ketoacidosis is a fruity breath odor and Kussmaul's respirations. **(M-S)**

▶ A sign of diabetic ketoacidosis is ketones, which are the byproduct of fat metabolism that occurs when the body can't use glucose as an energy source and breaks down fat as a substitute. **(M-S)**

▶ The only insulin that can be given I.V. is regular insulin. **(M-S)**

▶ Regular insulin is routinely given 30 minutes before meals. **(M-S)**

▶ The best indication that the mother is bonding with her baby is that she talks to the baby and touches him. **(MAT)**

▶ If the new mother is afraid to provide care to her newborn because she doesn't feel she has the skills, the nurse should provide the care by demonstrating the techniques to the mother and helping the mother to provide the care. **(MAT)**

▶ If the infant is experiencing symptoms of narcotics withdrawal, the nurse should reduce environmental noises and stimulation. **(PED)**

▶ Signs of heroin withdrawal in the newborn include hyperactivity, irritability, and high-pitched crying. **(MAT)**

▶ Infantile anxiety is manifested by frequent crying. **(PSY)**

▶ According to the self-help group Alcoholics Anonymous, the first step toward recovering is admitting that you're an alcoholic and the first step in treatment of the alcoholic is detoxification. **(PSY)**

▶ Inflammation of the eyes is a frequent symptom in the person who recently smoked marijuana. **(PSY)**

▶ Although marijuana isn't known for its addictive qualities, use often leads to experimentation with other drugs and is known to cause apathy and suppress motivation. **(PSY)**

▶ After the death of a loved one, the nurse should allow the family to be with the remains; doing so promotes the reality of their loss and provides an opportunity for the grieving process to begin. **(FND)**

▶ The best indication that the patient with nephrotic syndrome is beginning to respond to the corticosteroid therapy is urinary output. **(M-S)**

▶ The best method for preventing blood clots after surgery is ambulation. **(M-S)**

▶ Adverse effects of aminophyllines include restlessness, irritability, tachycardia, hypertension, and insomnia. **(M-S)**

▶ The postmenopausal woman should do breast self-examination on the same day of each month, such as the first day of the month or the day of the month of her birthday. **(M-S)**

▶ Antibiotics are ineffective in the treatment of viruses. **(M-S)**

▶ When a change in the patient's condition indicates a need to notify the doctor, the nurse should first assess the patient so that she can provide accurate and complete information to the doctor. **(FND)**

▶ Persistent use of a nasal decongestant can cause "rebound phenomenon," which results in the congestion becoming worse. **(M-S)**

▶ Having a blood relative with breast cancer increases the patient's risk of developing the cancer. **(M-S)**

▶ Fibrocystic lesions observed on X-ray in benign fibrocystic disease become larger and tender just before menses. **(M-S)**

▶ Cancerous tumors tend to be irregularly shaped and attached to surrounding tissue so that the tumors don't move freely. **(M-S)**

▶ A baseline mammogram should be done between the ages of 35 and 39; routine mammograms should be done every 1 to 2 years between ages 40 and 49 and annually at age 50 and older. **(M-S)**

▶ As part of self-examination of her breasts, a woman should observe her breasts for asymmetry by standing before a mirror with her bra removed and her arms above her head. **(M-S)**

▶ The pads of the four fingertips should be used in examining the breasts. **(M-S)**

▶ The patient should be instructed that one of the methods for examining the breasts is to palpate in small circles from the outer margins toward the nipples. **(M-S)**

▶ The patient scheduled for a mammogram should be instructed to not use underarm deodorant, body powder, or ointment; because these substances could cause an artifact in the film. **(M-S)**

▶ The drug of choice for treating status epilepticus is diazepam (Valium) I.V. **(M-S)**

▶ Oral hygiene is extremely important to the patient on phenytoin sodium (Dilantin). **(M-S)**

▶ Following a head injury, clear fluid in the ears (cerebrospinal fluid) indicates that the meninges may have been injured. **(M-S)**

▶ When it's essential to move the patient with a possible head and neck injury, immobilize the head and neck and move them as a single unit. **(M-S)**

▶ The patient with a head injury should be maintained in a supine position with his head slightly elevated to reduce intracranial pressure and promote venous return. **(M-S)**

▶ The best indicator of increasing intracranial pressure is a deteriorating level of consciousness; another indication is abnormal pupillary response such as dilation when a light is shined into the eye. **(M-S)**

▶ The patient on mannitol should have a catheter because of the osmotic effect of the drug, since the osmotic effect causes increased urination. **(M-S)**

▶ Adverse effects associated with mannitol therapy include dehydration, electrolyte imbalance, and diarrhea. **(M-S)**

▶ The primary nursing intervention for the child admitted to the hospital in a sickle cell crisis is relieving pain. **(PED)**

▶ Because the child in a sickle cell crisis is prone to dehydration, he should be offered favorite fluids, such as ice pops and gelatins. **(PED)**

▶ If both parents have the sickle cell trait (both parents are heterozygous), there is a 25% chance that an offspring would be born with sickle cell disease. **(PED)**

▶ The infant with acquired immunodeficiency syndrome often presents with thrush, mouth sores, and severe diaper rash. **(PED)**

▶ A suggested cause of atopic dermatitis is an allergic reaction. **(M-S)**

▶ The treatment for dermatitis is often directed at relieving pruritus (itching). **(M-S)**

▶ The most common colloid bath used to treat the irritated, itchy skin of the infant with eczema is a mixture of baking soda and cornstarch in tepid water. **(PED)**

▶ Always suspect abuse if the child's injuries are inconsistent with his medical history and his wounds are in various stages of healing. **(PED)**

▶ When the child sustains a head injury, the parents should be instructed to assess the child for headaches and vomiting and to awaken the child every 4 hours to evaluate the difficulty in arousing the child. **(PED)**

▶ Pinworms should be suspected if the child experiences anal itching, especially at night. **(PED)**

▶ The best site for assessing the pulse of the child up to age 5 is the point of maximal impulse (apical pulse). **(PED)**

▶ The nurse should teach the parent to place the infant in an upright position and to use a rubber-tipped medicine dropper to administer oral medication. **(PED)**

▶ The child with hemophilia shouldn't be given products containing aspirin. **(PED)**

▶ Elbow restraints should be used to restrain the upper extremities of the infant who had a cleft lip repair.   **(PED)**

▶ The toddler is developing autonomy when he frequently responds "no" to his parents' requests for him to do something.   **(PED)**

▶ The child's fear and anxiety about a new procedure may be minimized by allowing the child, when appropriate, to handle the equipment.   **(PED)**

▶ Painful procedures shouldn't be performed in the child's hospital room; the child may come to view the room as a "torture chamber."   **(PED)**

▶ A sign of the child's severe reaction to prolonged hospitalization is ignoring his parents.   **(PED)**

▶ The nurse should encourage the parents to sleep in the room and participate in the care of the child to counter the effects of prolonged hospitalization.   **(PED)**

▶ A significant finding in assessing the parent's potential for child abuse is the fact that the parent was abused as a child.   **(PED)**

▶ When treating any person who is accused of a "crime against nature," sexual abuse, or child abuse, the nurse should maintain a nonjudgmental attitude.   **(PSY)**

▶ Allowing the mother to provide basic care for her newborn infant promotes bonding.   **(MAT)**

▶ *Reflecting* is a communicating process in which the person responds to the spoken word as well as the feeling associated with the message.   **(PSY)**

▶ Noisy respirations indicate that a tracheostomy needs suctioning.   **(M-S)**

▶ Before suctioning the patient, the nurse should provide 100% oxygen for 1 to 2 minutes.   **(M-S)**

▶ Wounds should be cleaned from the center to the outer edges to prevent transferring microorganisms from outside to inside the wound.   **(FND)**

▶ Hearing aids amplify sound waves so that the wearer can hear sounds better.   **(FND)**

▶ A common complaint of the patient with a retinal detachment is seeing a veil-like curtain in the visual field as well as flashes of light.   **(M-S)**

▶ Medication is normally not administered in bottle-feedings because the infant may not drink the entire contents of the bottle. **(PED)**

▶ The child in Bryant's traction shouldn't have a trapeze attached to the bed. **(PED)**

▶ The pregnant woman's urine test that's positive for albumin indicates the need for further assessment. **(MAT)**

▶ The maternity patient admitted to labor and delivery wouldn't normally receive an enema if she has vaginal bleeding. **(MAT)**

▶ Falling blood pressure, increased pulse, and increased respirations are all signs of impending shock in the postoperative patient. **(M-S)**

▶ Following a transurethral prostatic resection, the patient should be encouraged to drink large amounts of fluid to keep urine diluted and prevent blood clots from forming in the urine and obstructing the catheter. **(M-S)**

▶ If the patient is fully dilated and her cervix is 100% effaced, the patient is entering the second stage of labor. **(MAT)**

▶ One ounce is equal to 30 ml. **(FND)**

▶ The presence of a skin rash indicates that the patient may be experiencing a reaction to penicillin; therefore, the nurse should withhold the medication and notify the doctor. **(M-S)**

▶ To promote healthy elimination, adults should drink 1,500 ml of fluid a day and consume a regular diet that includes adequate amounts of fruits and vegetables. **(M-S)**

▶ To minimize discomfort when administering an I.M. injection into the dorsogluteal site, have the patient position his toes inward. **(FND)**

▶ Before administering influenza vaccine, the nurse should ask the patient if he's allergic to eggs or egg products. **(M-S)**

▶ The adult patient with a high fever should receive between 2,500 and 3,000 ml of fluid a day if he has no preexisting cardiovascular or kidney diseases. **(M-S)**

▶ A tepid bath is used to enhance body heat loss. **(FND)**

▶ The water temperature of a tepid bath should be 80° to 90° F (26.7° to 32.2° C). **(FND)**

▶ If the patient begins shivering or has chills, a tepid bath should be discontinued. **(FND)**

▶ The nurse should report an elevated temperature in the patient undergoing dialysis. **(M-S)**

▶ A suprapubic cystostomy tube is surgically inserted directly into the bladder and should have a urine flow consistent with the patient's routine urine output. **(M-S)**

▶ The adult patient with urolithiasis should receive 2,500 ml of fluid daily, ambulate frequently, and have his urine strained to harvest any stones that pass. **(M-S)**

▶ The patient undergoing extracorporeal shock wave lithotripsy usually has the lower half of his body submerged in water or has his body surrounded by fluid-filled bags and is given a preprocedural medication to reduce discomfort. **(M-S)**

▶ A consistent finding of the patient with benign prostatic hyperplasia is nocturia, hesitation on urination, a decrease in force of urinary stream, and dribbling. **(M-S)**

▶ Fertilization usually takes place in the fallopian tubes. **(MAT)**

▶ The size of the woman's breasts has no effect on her ability to breast-feed or provide adequate nutrition for her nursing infant. **(MAT)**

▶ The size of the true pelvis in comparison to the size of the fetus's head (cephalopelvic ratio) is one factor that may determine whether the maternity patient can deliver vaginally. **(MAT)**

▶ The 3- to 4-month-old infant in a prone position should be able to lift his head 45 to 90 degrees. **(PED)**

▶ If the infant pushes medication out of his mouth because of the extrusion reflex, the nurse should scoop it up and return it to the infant's mouth. **(PED)**

▶ New foods should be introduced to the 4- or 5-month-old infant one food at a time for approximately 1 week each to identify food allergies. **(PED)**

▶ Carotenosis is occasionally seen in infants being fed orange-colored vegetables such as carrots. **(PED)**

▶ Home water heaters shouldn't be set above 120° F (48.9° C). **(FND)**

▶ A high concentration of oxygen administered to the premature infant can cause retrolental fibroplasia and result in blindness. **(PED)**

▶ In an adolescent, the tell-tale signs of suicidal intention include loss of a significant friend, loss of a friend to suicide, a change in appearance, a decreased interest in activities that used to bring pleasure, a loss of interest in school, increased substance abuse, suicide notes, fascination with death, decreased appetite, and changes in hygiene. **(PSY)**

▶ Bladder training is usually easier to accomplish than bowel training and should be started at 18 to 24 months. **(PED)**

▶ In treating the child with impetigo, local and systemic antibiotics are normally used concomitantly, and fingernails are trimmed to prevent scratching. **(PED)**

▶ The best position for the child who is having a lumbar puncture is the side-lying position with the knees drawn up. **(PED)**

▶ Air leaking into surrounding tissue at the insertion site of a chest tube can result in subcutaneous emphysema. **(M-S)**

▶ To be more comfortable, the patient should void before having a pelvic examination. **(M-S)**

▶ A lithotomy position is preferred for performing a pelvic examination. **(FND)**

▶ If a lithotomy position can't be used for a pelvic examination because the patient has a preexisting condition such as multiple sclerosis, elevate the patient's hips on a pillow. **(FND)**

▶ Breakthrough bleeding often occurs during the early phase of oral contraceptive use. **(MAT)**

▶ A woman shouldn't douche for several days before a Papanicolaou test. **(M-S)**

▶ The patient should be instructed to perform a breast self-examination while taking a shower. **(M-S)**

▶ A blood pressure cuff bladder should cover at least two-thirds of the limb at midpoint and should be as wide as 40% midlimb circumference. **(FND)**

▶ The organ that usually sustains damage from hypertension is the eye. **(M-S)**

▶ Administration of diuretics in the morning minimizes disruption of sleep for urination. **(M-S)**

▶ Bananas, oranges, nectarines, and cantaloupe are good sources of potassium. **(FND)**

▶ Cholesterol is animal fat that attaches to the intimal layer of arteries and enlarges to form plaque that occludes the passageway of the vessels, causing atherosclerosis. **(M-S)**

▶ An adverse effect of nicotinic acid tablets used to lower triglyceride levels is flushing of the skin. **(M-S)**

▶ Adverse effects of colestipol (Colestid), an antihyperlipidemic drug, are constipation and abdominal pain and distention. **(M-S)**

▶ If, during a stress electrocardiogram, the patient develops chest pain, dangerous cardiac rhythm changes, or significant elevation of blood pressure, the test should be stopped. **(M-S)**

▶ Adverse effects of nitroglycerine tablets include headache, flushing, and dizziness. **(M-S)**

▶ If a food has 4 g of protein, 28 g of fat, and 62 g of carbohydrates, the number of calories is 516; protein and carbohydrates each have 4 calories per gram and fat has 9 calories per gram. **(FND)**

▶ Dizziness and vertigo are common adverse effects of the vasodilating drug isosorbide dinitrate (Isordil), which is used in the prolonged treatment of angina; these effects may be minimized by lowering the dosage or instructing the patient to take the medication at night before going to sleep. **(M-S)**

▶ Quite often the best nursing intervention for the anxious patient is simply to allow the patient to express his anxiety. **(PSY)**

▶ In communicating with the anxious patient, use short simple sentences. **(PSY)**

▶ Avoidance is the most common defense mechanism used by patients who have a phobia. **(PSY)**

▶ Art therapy is a therapeutic technique that may enable a person to share a thought too painful to discuss. **(PSY)**

▶ Any person who survives a catastrophic event or out-of-the-normal human experience is at risk for posttraumatic stress disorder. **(PSY)**

▶ Unless otherwise directed, the solution used to irrigate an indwelling urinary catheter is normal saline. **(FND)**

▶ A characteristic of obstructive jaundice is dark brown urine. **(M-S)**

▶ Dark urine occurs when the kidneys instead of the intestinal tract serve as the method of excreting bilirubin. **(M-S)**

▶ The desired safety outcome for the patient with osteoporosis is preventing injuries from falls. **(FND)**

▶ Before providing a bolus feeding via a gastric tube, the residual stomach content should be checked so gastric feedings will be held if there is more than 100 ml remaining from the previous feeding. **(M-S)**

▶ Following a gastric feeding, the gastric tube should be irrigated with water and the head of the bed should be elevated. **(FND)**

▶ Patients with gastric ulcers generally report that discomfort goes away after they eat food. **(M-S)**

▶ A positive result in occult blood test of the feces indicates bleeding in the GI tract. **(M-S)**

▶ Antibiotics such as tetracycline are administered to patients with peptic ulcers to eliminate *Helicobacter pylori,* bacteria that deplete gastric mucus. **(M-S)**

▶ A sign of a perforated ulcer includes abdominal rigidity and pain. **(M-S)**

▶ The method for determining proper placement of a gastric sump tube is to instill a bolus of air, then listen for a whooshing sound. **(FND)**

▶ To ensure that the patient performs postoperative procedures necessary for his recovery, the nurse should first alleviate pain through teaching the patient positioning, splinting, or controlled breathing or by administering prescribed analgesics. **(M-S)**

▶ Water used to irrigate a gastric tube should be recorded as intake on the intake and output record. **(FND)**

▶ The patient at risk for dumping syndrome is taught to consume a diet low in carbohydrates and to avoid fluids during meals. **(M-S)**

▶ The patient who had a partial gastrectomy should be taught to eat small meals and to lie down for a short period after eating to delay gastric emptying. **(M-S)**

▶ Absence of free hydrochloric acid suggests stomach cancer. **(M-S)**

▶ When inserting a nasogastric tube preoperatively, having the patient place his chin to his chest will facilitate passage of the tube down the esophagus and away from the trachea. **(FND)**

▶ Low intermittent suction is best for single-lumen nasogastric tubes. **(FND)**

▶ Low continuous suction is best for vented, or double-lumen, nasogastric tubes. **(FND)**

► The patient who is undergoing nasogastric suctioning should receive nothing by mouth because the fluid instilled will be suctioned out of the stomach, further depleting the electrolytes and causing an imbalance. **(FND)**

► There are 1,000 mcg in 1 mg. **(FND)**

► There are 62.5 mg in 1 grain. **(FND)**

► Concentrated urine is one of the first signs of dehydration. **(M-S)**

► A trochanter roll is used to maintain the hip in a neutral position and prevent external rotation. **(FND)**

► A footboard is used to prevent plantar flexion and foot drop deformity. **(FND)**

► One teaspoon equals 5 ml; 1 tbs equals 15 ml. **(FND)**

► When administering solid medication and cough syrup at the same sitting, administer the cough syrup last. **(FND)**

► The best method for aiding expectoration of pulmonary secretions is increased fluid intake to thin secretions. **(M-S)**

► After obtaining a sputum specimen, provide oral hygiene care. **(FND)**

► The most common characteristic of pleurisy is a sharp, stabbing pain on inspiration. **(M-S)**

► There is a relationship between genital warts caused by the human papillomavirus and the development of cancer in the vulva, vagina, and cervix. **(M-S)**

► The patient should use a condom containing the spermicide nonoxynol-9 to reduce the spread of human immunodeficiency virus. **(M-S)**

► Oral contraceptives are best taken at approximately the same time each day, preferably in the evening. **(M-S)**

► In the patient taking oral contraceptives, smoking increases the risk of developing blood clots. **(M-S)**

► Following a vasectomy, the patient should use an additional method of birth control for 6 weeks; he should have a zero sperm count before considering himself sterile. **(M-S)**

► Complications of percutaneous transluminal coronary angioplasty include chest pain, abnormal cardiac rhythms, and bleeding from the operative site. **(M-S)**

▶ Bleeding is the most common adverse reaction associated with thrombolytic drug therapy. **(M-S)**

▶ The best method for opening the airway of the unconscious patient is chin lift and head tilt. **(M-S)**

▶ After successful cardiopulmonary resuscitation, the nurse should place the patient in a side-lying position. **(M-S)**

▶ A sudden increase in energy in the maternity patient is associated with "nesting instinct" and indicates approaching labor. **(MAT)**

▶ During the latent phase of the first stage of labor, the maternity patient is encouraged to drink fluids to prevent dehydration. **(MAT)**

▶ The fetal heart rate should be assessed every 30 minutes during the latent phase of labor, every 15 minutes in the active phase, and every 5 minutes in the transition phase. **(MAT)**

▶ Epidural anesthesia can be performed at anytime during labor; however, it's usually given when the primigravida is dilated 5 to 6 cm and the multigravida is dilated 3 to 4 cm. **(MAT)**

▶ In assessing uterine contractions, the nurse should palpate the fundus of the uterus just above the umbilicus because the contractions are strongest at this location. **(MAT)**

▶ The first action the nurse should take upon noting that the membranes have ruptured is to assess fetal heart tones. **(MAT)**

▶ After the rupture of membranes, the patient's temperature should be assessed every hour because of the increased risk of infection. **(MAT)**

▶ An episiotomy prevents laceration and damage to the perineum and speeds up the delivery process. **(MAT)**

▶ To insert a vaginal suppository, the patient should be in a lying position with knees flexed. **(MAT)**

▶ Vaginal suppositories are best administered at bedtime; a recumbent position aids in retaining the medication. **(FND)**

▶ Yeast is present in the intestinal tract and is spread into the vagina by wiping from the rectum to the vagina; therefore, teach the patient to wipe from front to back. **(FND)**

▶ Infertility is commonly caused by pelvic inflammatory disease. **(M-S)**

▶ The nurse should walk behind and slightly to the side of the patient using a walker. **(FND)**

▶ The best time to do postural drainage is in the morning. **(FND)**

▶ The only way to prevent contractures is exercise. **(FND)**

▶ Following a myocardial infarction, nursing action is directed at providing rest to the heart muscle by providing bed rest, oxygen, pain relief, and a bedside commode. **(M-S)**

▶ Following cataract extraction, intraocular tension should be minimized by encouraging the patient to rest his eyes by using eye patches, avoid reading until cleared by the physician, avoid straining to defecate, avoid bending at the waist, and avoid lying with the affected eye dependent. **(M-S)**

▶ Stress incontinence can be relieved to a certain degree by using Kegel exercises to strengthen the pubococcygeal muscles. **(M-S)**

▶ To determine if the patient is adapting to changes created by illness or injury, assess whether he acknowledges the deficit and chooses a level of activity that appropriately challenges his physical and mental capabilities. **(FND)**

▶ During a spinal tap, the patient must remain motionless and avoid any movement or coughing. **(M-S)**

▶ After the patient has a cholecystectomy, the nurse should clamp the T tube when the patient eats. **(M-S)**

▶ Exercising the legs helps prevent venous stasis and the formation of venous thrombosis. **(M-S)**

▶ Delirium tremens most often manifests as progressive deterioration of mental processes and orientation to person, place, and time. **(PSY)**

▶ For the patient with Alzheimer's disease, the room should be brightly lit during the daytime. **(M-S)**

▶ If the patient receiving an enema complains that he is unable to retain the fluid any longer, clamp the tubing and instruct him to take deep breaths. **(FND)**

▶ The elderly client has a decreased need for calories. **(M-S)**

▶ Use of an over-the-bed trapeze is contraindicated for the patient with a ruptured lumbar disk. **(M-S)**

▶ The patient shouldn't use makeup, including lipstick and powder, before surgery; it could interfere with visual assessment of the patient. **(M-S)**

▶ In treating the burn patient, the priority concern is assessment of airway function. **(M-S)**

▶ To conserve the energy of the premature infant, the nurse should cluster nursing care activities. **(PED)**

▶ Following insertion of tympanostomy tubes in the child, the parent should be instructed to have the child wear earplugs when bathing. **(PED)**

▶ The most common adverse effects of isoniazid are peripheral neuritis, hepatitis, and hypersensitivity. **(M-S)**

▶ When the patient is on isoniazid, aspartate aminotransferase and alanine aminotransferase levels should be monitored. **(M-S)**

▶ Sputum cultures on three consecutive mornings must be negative for the patient with tuberculosis to be considered no longer infectious. **(M-S)**

▶ Following removal of a catheter, dribbling may occur because of a weakened urinary sphincter. **(M-S)**

▶ The respiratory status of the patient should be assessed before administering meperidine hydrochloride (Demerol), which is a central nervous system depressant. **(M-S)**

▶ Tomato juice contains a high amount of vitamin C, which promotes wound healing. **(FND)**

▶ When questioning a patient, the nurse should go from general to specific, for example, "Are you experiencing any pain?" followed by "Could you tell me the location of your pain?" **(FND)**

▶ The first symptom of tracheal edema secondary to trauma associated with bronchoscopy is dyspnea. **(M-S)**

▶ A chest tube is inserted to drain blood and other fluids and to reestablish and maintain negative pressure. **(M-S)**

▶ Risk factors for coronary artery disease include obesity, diet high in saturated fats, and increasing amounts of stress. **(M-S)**

▶ During the immediate postamputation phase, pain medication is the treatment of choice. **(M-S)**

▶ The best source of information regarding a patient's illness is the patient himself. **(FND)**

▶ The goal of performing surgical preparation is to reduce the total number of bacteria. **(M-S)**

▶ If the patient has no signs of dehydration but his oral mucous membranes are dry, he's breathing through his mouth instead of his nose. **(FND)**

▶ A newly applied plaster cast normally dries within 24 hours and dries from the outside to the inside. **(FND)**

▶ Aminophylline relaxes the smooth muscles of the bronchi and relieves bronchospasms. **(M-S)**

▶ Before amniocentesis, the patient should empty her bladder. **(MAT)**

▶ Protein is restricted in patients with severe renal impairment because they are unable to eliminate nitrogen, a waste product of protein metabolism. **(M-S)**

▶ Vitamin D is known as "the sunshine vitamin." **(FND)**

▶ Orange and green vegetables are the primary source of vitamin A. **(FND)**

▶ Clothing that becomes wet in a mist (moist) tent should be changed. **(FND)**

▶ The mist in a moist tent should never be so dense that it obstructs the view of the patient's breathing pattern. **(FND)**

▶ The toenails of a diabetic patient should be cut and filed straight across. **(FND)**

▶ Night blindness is associated with vitamin A deficiency. **(FND)**

▶ Following a liver biopsy, nursing care is directed at minimizing the risk of hemorrhage. **(M-S)**

▶ If the patient complains of incomplete emptying after a colostomy irrigation, the nurse should irrigate the colostomy with normal saline and suggest a morning evacuation. **(M-S)**

▶ The newborn who has hydrocephalus should have his position changed every 1 to 2 hours. **(PED)**

▶ When feeding the infant who has had a cleft lip repair, place the infant in an upright position to facilitate swallowing, burping, and retention of formula or breast milk. **(PED)**

▶ Before putting antiembolism stockings on the patient, the nurse should have the patient lie down with the feet elevated for 20 to 30 minutes. **(FND)**

▶ When performing a gastric gavage feeding, the nurse should place the patient in an upright position to minimize the risk of reflux. **(FND)**

▶ An enteric-coated tablet shouldn't be crushed; it's designed to be dissolved in the GI tract. **(M-S)**

▶ The nurse should walk slightly in front of the blind patient. **(FND)**

▶ To help a patient with poor vision locate his food on the tray, refer to times on a clock (for instance, "Your potatoes are at 12 o'clock; your bread is at 3 o'clock, and your steak is at 6 o'clock.") **(FND)**

▶ When weighing the patient with anorexia nervosa, the nurse should have the patient step backward onto the scale while guiding her to ensure her safety. **(M-S)**

▶ After administering ear medication, maintain the child in a side-lying position for 2 to 3 minutes so the medication reaches the middle ear and ear drum. **(PED)**

▶ Hyperpyrexia puts the child at an increased risk of seizures. **(M-S)**

▶ The treatment protocol for acute leukemia involves three phases: induction (the patient receives chemotherapy), consolidation (modified course of chemotherapy), and maintenance (small doses of chemotherapy every 3 to 4 weeks). **(M-S)**

▶ Before attempting to teach the patient any procedure or task, assess the patient's willingness to learn and his current level of knowledge. **(FND)**

▶ Clear liquids refer to liquids that can be seen through. **(FND)**

▶ The purpose of administering a cleansing enema before a barium enema is to facilitate visualization of the colon. **(FND)**

▶ Thiazides are potassium-depleting diuretics, and the patient taking them should increase his oral intake of potassium. **(M-S)**

▶ The nurse should report a prolonged clotting time to the doctor; normally, slow clotting results in postponement of surgery. **(M-S)**

▶ Three cellular products that assist the body in its fight against infection or invasion are interferon, lymphokines, and interleukins. **(M-S)**

▶ The daily dose of digoxin is 0.125 to 0.5 mg daily. **(M-S)**

▶ Furosemide (Lasix) is a potassium-sparing diuretic. **(M-S)**

▶ A sign that heart failure is resolving is increased urine output.
(M-S)

▶ Risk for "body image disturbance" is a diagnosis for the female with Cushing's syndrome; she's at risk for developing malelike characteristics (known as masculinization). **(M-S)**

▶ The first indication of an impending thyroid crisis in the patient with Graves' disease is an elevation of temperature over baseline.
(M-S)

▶ A sign of Graves' disease (hyperthyroidism) is exophthalmus (bulging eyes). **(M-S)**

▶ A drug used in the treatment of hyperthyroidism is thionamides (propylthiouracil). **(M-S)**

▶ Thionamides should be stored in a light-resistant container and taken at the prescribed time throughout the day (normally every 8 hours). **(M-S)**

▶ Following a complete or partial parathyroidectomy, the patient should consume a diet high in calcium. **(M-S)**

▶ Calcium gluconate and calcium chloride I.V. are the drugs of choice for treating tetany associated with hypothyroidism. **(M-S)**

▶ A bronzelike pigmentation of the skin is associated with Addison's disease. **(M-S)**

▶ Patients with Addison's disease should select foods high in sodium, such as cheese, milk, and processed (canned) foods. **(M-S)**

▶ Extreme stress, salt depletion, infection, trauma, and extremes in temperature place the patient with Addison's disease at increased risk for an addisonian crisis. **(M-S)**

▶ Addisonian crisis is manifested by severe hypotension and requires the administration of I.V. cortisol to reverse the signs and symptoms associated with the crisis. **(M-S)**

▶ A parathyroid tumor normally causes a shift of calcium from the bones to the blood and results in renal calculi and leg cramps. **(M-S)**

▶ A decrease in bone mass secondary to a loss of calcium from the bones places the patient at increased risk for pathologic fractures. **(M-S)**

▶ The normal fetal heart rate is 120 to 160 beats per minute (including the rate during contractions). **(MAT)**

▶ The fundus should be at the level of the symphysis pubis in the patient in her 12th week of pregnancy. **(MAT)**

▶ The maternity patient without any complications should be seen monthly for the first 28 weeks, every 2 weeks up to 36 weeks, and then weekly until delivery. **(MAT)**

▶ When lifting the patient's legs to place them in a lithotomy position, both legs should be lifted at the same time. **(FND)**

▶ Signs of corneal transplant rejection include loss of vision, redness, and photosensitivity. **(M-S)**

▶ Even if the patient taking interferon for multiple sclerosis develops anorexia and nausea, the medication needs to be administered; try smaller, more frequent meals. **(M-S)**

▶ Mirrors should be removed from the room of the patient with facial burns until he's counseled regarding the disfigurement. **(M-S)**

▶ A consistent finding in patients with multiple sclerosis is that hot weather and hot water increase weakness. **(M-S)**

▶ When injecting a medication into the patient who has received a previous injection, don't use a site that is closer than 1″ (2.5 cm) to a previous site. **(FND)**

▶ The size of a needle for a small to medium adult is 1½″ (3.8 cm) for I.M. injections. **(FND)**

▶ The mitral valve is located between the left atrium and the left ventricle. **(FND)**

▶ Clubbing of digits is a consistent finding in adults and children with chronic cardiopulmonary diseases. **(M-S)**

▶ An elevated temperature, which inhibits and destroys pathogens, is the body's mechanism for fighting infections. **(M-S)**

▶ A sign of pericarditis is a friction rub, which has a grating or leathery sound. **(M-S)**

▶ Signs of diabetes insipidus are polyuria, a craving for cold water, and a urine specific gravity of less than 1.005. **(M-S)**

▶ Morning urine is usually the most concentrated and is best for routine urinalysis. **(FND)**

▶ A sign of acromegaly is enlarged hands. **(M-S)**

▶ A water-deprivation test is used to aid in diagnosing diabetes insipidus; even when deprived of water, the kidneys can't concentrate urine. **(M-S)**

▶ During the oliguric phase of renal failure, the patient is given fluid only equal to the amount of urine output. **(M-S)**

▶ When the patient is on strict intake and output, the amount of fluid permitted is distributed throughout the day (for example, 50% is given during the day shift, 30% during the evening shift, and 20% during the night shift). **(FND)**

▶ If the patient in renal failure is administered a "fluid challenge" of 500 ml of I.V. fluids, it's essential to monitor for signs of heart failure and pulmonary edema. **(M-S)**

▶ If the patient on fluid restriction complains of being thirsty, hard candy may be used to provide a measure of relief. **(M-S)**

▶ The autistic child responds to his parents and others with indifference. **(PED)**

▶ Autistic children often display bizarre repetitive body movements. **(PED)**

▶ The autistic child needs to be protected from self-harm, such as head banging and self-biting. **(PED)**

▶ Keep the environment of the autistic child consistent and avoid changing routines. **(PED)**

▶ School-age children are normally told about medical procedures several days to a week before they occur, while toddlers are usually told just before the event occurs (normally no more than a day), and infants are told just as the event happens. **(PED)**

▶ Before discontinuing an indwelling urinary catheter that has been in place for an extended time, the nurse should clamp the tubing and allow the bladder to expand several times. **(FND)**

▶ The child with croup shouldn't be given cough suppressants; suppressing the cough may worsen the child's respiratory status. **(PED)**

▶ Total parenteral nutrition should be stored in the refrigerator and removed 30 to 60 minutes before delivery; chilled solution can cause hypothermia. **(FND)**

▶ The primary purpose in providing skin care at the insertion site of skeletal pins is to protect the bone from osteomyelitis. **(M-S)**

▶ Pill-rolling tremor is a classic sign of Parkinson's disease. **(M-S)**

▶ Respiratory distress is a manifestation of fat embolism, which occurs 24 to 48 hours after the fracture of a long bone. **(M-S)**

▶ The patient's bed bath should proceed in this order: face, neck, arms, hands, chest, abdomen, back, legs, and perineum. **(FND)**

▶ To break the suction of the nursing infant, the mother should insert her finger into the corner of the infant's mouth or gently press his chin downward. **(MAT)**

▶ Following a percutaneous bladder aspiration, the patient's urine may be a slight pink color; frank bleeding should be reported to the doctor. **(M-S)**

▶ A Bradford frame is used for children who must be immobilized for a long time. **(PED)**

▶ Beriberi disease, which is manifested by profound weakness, is a serious deficiency of vitamin B_1. **(M-S)**

▶ The nurse should use a Z-track method of administering injectable forms of iron. **(FND)**

▶ The patient who receives an organ transplant must take an immunosuppressant drug for life. **(M-S)**

▶ A sign of a congenital hip dislocation is an Ortolani's click, which is heard on abduction of the neonate's leg on the affected side. **(PED)**

▶ Treatment for congenital hip dislocation is a Pavlik's harness or the use of two or three diapers to maintain the leg in abduction. **(M-S)**

▶ The first sign of a pressure ulcer is redness, then blanching. **(M-S)**

▶ Red tissue that blanches should be massaged and preventive measures should be instituted to prevent an ulcer from forming. For example, increase the frequency of turning, ensure an adequate diet, maintain a clean and dry bed, and prevent shearing force, friction, and pressure injuries. **(M-S)**

▶ Signs of thalassemia major include pronounced bone hyperactivity, resulting in thickening of the cranium, and a Down syndrome appearance. **(M-S)**

▶ The neonate's head is typically 1″ (2 to 3 cm) larger than his chest. **(MAT)**

▶ "Birds of a feather flock together" and "Don't cry over spilled milk" are examples of proverbs used to assess the patient's ability to abstract. **(PSY)**

▶ The ability to abstract is compromised in schizophrenics, who often think in concrete terms; for example, the patient with schizophrenia might interpret "people who live in glass houses shouldn't throw stones" as "the stones will break the glass." **(PSY)**

▶ Possible allergic reactions to iodine dye include dyspnea, sweating, nausea, vomiting, and chills. **(M-S)**

▶ The major complications of paracentesis are hypovolemia and shock from fluid drainage and fluid shift. **(M-S)**

▶ Otitis media is common in the infant with a cleft palate. **(PED)**

▶ Clinical manifestations of malabsorption syndrome are weight loss, muscle wasting, bloating, and steatorrhea. **(M-S)**

▶ The patient receiving chemotherapy is placed in reverse isolation. **(M-S)**

▶ A fever in the first 24 hours following delivery is more likely the result of dehydration than infection. **(MAT)**

▶ In the patient recovering from tonsillectomy, frequent swallowing suggests hemorrhage. **(M-S)**

▶ Two common manifestations of systemic lupus erythematosus are early morning stiffness and facial erythema in a butterfly pattern. **(M-S)**

▶ Hypovolemia is the most common, and the most fatal, complication of acute pancreatitis. **(M-S)**

▶ When instilling eye ointment and eyedrops into the same eye, administer the eyedrops first. **(FND)**

▶ The infant with gastroesophageal reflux should receive formula thickened with cereal. **(PED)**

▶ The child with measles or chickenpox should be put in isolation. **(PED)**

▶ Greenstick fractures are the most common type of fractures in children. **(PED)**

▶ The nurse's role regarding a patient's will is to record in his health record that he made a will and to document his current mental status. **(FND)**

▶ Fetal alcohol syndrome presents in the first 24 hours after birth. **(MAT)**

▶ The infant's respiratory rate and apical pulse should be counted for 1 minute. **(PED)**

▶ The first cardinal sign of toxic shock syndrome is the rapid onset of a high fever. **(M-S)**

▶ Frothy, blood-tinged sputum is a sign of pulmonary edema. **(M-S)**

▶ A tuning fork is used in the Rinne or Weber test to assess for sensory or conductive hearing loss. **(M-S)**

▶ The fulminating form of hepatitis resembles acute liver failure and may result in death. **(M-S)**

▶ Insulin promotes conversion of fatty acids to fat, regulates the rate that carbohydrates are used by cells for energy, and stimulates protein synthesis. **(M-S)**

▶ Delta hepatitis (hepatitis D) must coexist with hepatitis B. **(M-S)**

▶ Food and water intake aren't restricted before a thyroid function test. **(M-S)**

▶ After signing a consent form for a procedure, the patient makes a statement suggesting he doesn't understand the procedure, therefore indicating that he isn't informed. In such a case, the doctor should be notified of the patient's lack of understanding before the patient receives preprocedure medication. **(FND)**

▶ Children with hepatitis are usually anicteric. **(PED)**

▶ A normal healthy stoma appears bright red or pink, while a sustained dark color or paleness indicates compromised blood flow to the tissue. **(M-S)**

▶ A low-residue diet contains no fruits, vegetables, or whole grains or cereals. **(FND)**

▶ If a patient experiences a traumatic evisceration of the bowel, the nurse should cover the exposed bowel with sterile, saline-soaked gauze. **(M-S)**

▶ Following insertion of a Miller-Abbott intestinal tube, the patient should be ambulated. **(M-S)**

▶ The best position for irrigating a stoma is sitting on a toilet. **(FND)**

▶ One of the best methods for determining whether the patient's stool is impacted is digital examination. **(M-S)**

▶ Carbonated beverages tend to promote gas production and should be eliminated from the diet of the patient prone to tympanites. **(M-S)**

▶ The primary purpose of a sitz bath is comfort. **(FND)**

▶ The most common form of cirrhosis of the liver in the United States is Laënnec's cirrhosis secondary to alcohol abuse. **(M-S)**

▶ Spider angiomas are consistent findings of patients with Laënnec's cirrhosis and are manifested by central red bodies and radiating branches. **(M-S)**

▶ The bladder should be emptied before paracentesis. **(M-S)**

▶ Patients with Tourette's syndrome tend to make uncontrollable audible sounds or utter obscenities. **(M-S)**

▶ A sign of cystic fibrosis is salty-tasting skin. **(M-S)**

▶ A postoperative diet is usually clear liquids for the first 24 hours. **(M-S)**

▶ To reduce the risk of paralytic ileus, the patient who has had general anesthesia won't be given solid food until he has a return of bowel sounds. **(M-S)**

▶ A doll should be used as a teaching aid to strengthen the preschooler's understanding of a procedure. **(PED)**

▶ It's normal for a 4- or 5-year-old child to have an imaginary friend. **(PED)**

▶ The patient with systemic lupus erythematosus should be provided a calm environment, be protected from the sun, and should avoid the use of dusting powder. **(M-S)**

▶ Continuous bubbling is abnormal in a water-sealed chamber but normal in a suction-controlled chamber. **(FND)**

▶ If recapping a needle is unavoidable, the nurse should use the one-hand scoop method. **(FND)**

▶ Eyedrops are instilled in the lower conjunctival sac to prevent damaging the cornea. **(FND)**

▶ Constipation is an adverse reaction to antacids. **(M-S)**

▶ Hospice-care facilities provide care for terminally ill patients. **(FND)**

▶ Respite care provides temporary nursing care so that the primary caregiver has an opportunity to do other activities. **(FND)**

▶ Grunting on expiration, see-saw retractions, and nasal flaring are signs of respiratory distress in the infant. **(PED)**

▶ Liquid supplements should be offered between meals so that the supplements don't take the place of meals. **(FND)**

▶ Before performing a procedure on the adult, and even before bringing equipment to the bedside, the nurse should explain what is going to take place. **(FND)**

▶ The first action to take in resuscitation is establishing or maintaining an airway. **(M-S)**

▶ Acceptance of an alteration in body appearance is best indicated by the patient looking at, and even touching, the affected area. **(FND)**

▶ Dizziness, light-headedness, and nausea and vomiting are symptoms of supine hypotension syndrome, which is treated by having the patient turn to his left side and to explain the cause so that the patient can prevent a recurrence. **(M-S)**

▶ *Gravidity* is the number of pregnancies without regard to outcome. *Parity* is the number of pregnancies that reached viability (20+ weeks). Further clarification of obstetric data is made using a system referred to as **F/TPAL**:

F/T means full-term delivery at 38+ weeks.

P means preterm delivery between 20 and 37 weeks.

A means abortion or loss of fetus before 20 weeks.

L means number of children living (if a child has died, further explanation is needed to clarify the discrepancy in numbers). **(MAT)**

▶ *Parity* doesn't refer to the number of viable fetuses delivered, only to the number of deliveries. **(MAT)**

▶ The recommended iron supplement for the pregnant patient is 30 to 60 mg daily. **(MAT)**

▶ For early identification of genetic defects, chorionic villus sampling is done at 8 to 12 weeks of pregnancy. **(MAT)**

▶ Percutaneous umbilical blood sampling is a procedure in which a blood sample is obtained from the umbilical cord to evaluate for anemia, genetic defects, and blood incompatibility. **(MAT)**

▶ *Uterine atony* is the failure of the uterus to remain firmly contracted, and the major cause is a full bladder. **(MAT)**

▶ The caregiver should burp the infant before initiating feeding to expel any air in the stomach. **(PED)**

▶ In patients with mastitis, most authorities strongly encourage the continuation of breast-feeding both on the affected and on the unaffected side. **(MAT)**

▶ The ideal place to check skin turgor on the infant is on the abdomen. **(PED)**

▶ The lag between head movement and eye movement is referred to as doll's eye movement and is normal. **(M-S)**

▶ The most desirable diet for the infant up to age 6 months is breast milk. **(PED)**

▶ When accessing whether the infant is ready for the addition of solids to his diet, look for the following indicators: (1) the infant has doubled his weight, (2) the infant demands between 8 and 10 feedings in a 24-hour period, (3) the infant drinks more than 1 qt of formula per day; and (4) the infant always seems hungry. **(PED)**

▶ Solids are introduced to the infant in the following order: rice cereal, fruits, oatmeal, prepared vegetables, and meat. **(PED)**

▶ The hepatitis B vaccine is given within 48 hours of birth. **(MAT)**

▶ Hepatitis B immune globulin is given within 12 hours of birth. **(MAT)**

▶ HELLP syndrome is an unusual variation of pregnancy-induced hypertension; the acronym stands for *h*emolysis, *e*levated *l*iver enzymes, and *l*ow *p*latelets. **(MAT)**

▶ Maternal serum alpha-fetoprotein is detectable at 7 weeks and peaks in the 3rd trimester; high levels detected between the 16th and 18th week are associated with neural-tube defects. **(MAT)**

▶ An arrest of descent occurs when the fetus fails to descend through the pelvic cavity during labor; it's often associated with cephalopelvic disproportion, and cesarean intervention is required. **(MAT)**

▶ Third spacing of fluid is a shifting of fluid from the intravascular space to the interstitial space where it remains. **(FND)**

▶ *Thought broadcasting* is a type of delusion in which the person believes that his thoughts are being "broadcast for the world to hear." **(PSY)**

▶ Advise the patient on griseofulvin to maintain a high-fat diet, which enhances the secretion of bile. **(M-S)**

▶ Foods high in protein decrease the absorption of levodopa. **(M-S)**

▶ Cottage cheese, cream cheese, yogurt, and sour cream are permitted in the diet of the patient taking a monoamine oxidate inhibitor for depression. **(PSY)**

▶ Normal central venous pressure is 2 to 8 mm Hg or 5 to 10 cm H_2O.
(M-S)

▶ A decrease in central venous pressure indicates a fall in circulating fluid volume as seen in shock. **(M-S)**

▶ A rise in central venous pressure is associated with an increase in circulating fluid volume as seen in renal failure. **(M-S)**

▶ If a central venous pressure reading is to be obtained when the patient is on a ventilator, the reading should be taken at the end of the expiratory cycle. **(M-S)**

▶ To ensure an accurate baseline central venous pressure reading, the zero point of the transducer must be at the level of the right atrium. **(M-S)**

▶ Mönckeberg's arteriosclerosis is a condition of calcium deposits in the medial layer of the arterial walls. **(M-S)**

▶ CK-MB, an isoenzyme of creatine kinase specific to the heart, increases 4 to 6 hours after a myocardial infarction, peaks at 12 to 18 hours, and returns to normal in 3 to 4 days. **(M-S)**

▶ The patient who survives a myocardial infarction and is without any other cardiopathology normally requires 6 to 12 weeks for a full recovery. **(M-S)**

▶ Risk factors associated with embolism are increased blood viscosity, decreased circulation, prolonged bed rest, and increased blood coagulability. **(M-S)**

▶ Sexual intercourse with a known partner is normally resumed 4 to 8 weeks after a myocardial infarction. **(M-S)**

▶ The patient recovering from a myocardial infarction should avoid eating or drinking alcoholic beverages before engaging in sexual intercourse. **(M-S)**

▶ *Dependent edema* is an early sign of right-sided heart failure seen in the legs where increased capillary hydrostatic pressure overwhelms plasma protein and causes a shift of fluid from the capillary beds to the interstitial spaces. **(M-S)**

▶ The patient who has had supratentorial surgery should have the head of the bed elevated to 30 degrees. **(M-S)**

▶ An acid or ash diet acidifies urine. **(M-S)**

▶ Vitamin C and cranberry juice acidify urine. **(FND)**

▶ The patient taking ColBENEMID (probenecid with colchicine) for gout should be instructed to take the medication with food. **(M-S)**

▶ If wound dehiscence is suspected, lay the patient down, examine the wound, and monitor vital signs; report concerns or abnormal findings to the doctor. **(M-S)**

▶ Miotics such as pilocarpine are administered to the patient with acute glaucoma to increase the outflow of aqueous humor. **(M-S)**

▶ Zoster immune globulin is administered to the patient to stimulate immunity to varicella. **(M-S)**

▶ The most common symptoms associated with compartmental syndrome are pain not relieved by analgesics, loss of movement, loss of sensation, pain with passive movement, and lack of pulse. **(M-S)**

▶ To help the patient with multiple sclerosis relieve muscle spasms, administer lioresal (Baclofen) as ordered, assist the patient with a warm soothing bath, and teach him progressive relaxation techniques. **(M-S)**

▶ The patient with a cervical spine injury and impairment at C5 should be able to lift his shoulders and elbows partially, but he will have no sensation below the clavicle. **(M-S)**

▶ The patient with a cervical spine injury and impairment at C6 should be able to lift his shoulders, elbows, and wrists partially, but he will have no sensation below the clavicle except a little in his arms and thumbs. **(M-S)**

▶ The patient with a cervical spine injury and impairment at C7 should be able to lift his shoulders, elbows, wrists, and hands partially, but he will have no sensation below midchest. **(M-S)**

▶ Injuries to the spinal cord C3 and above may be fatal because of a loss of innervation to the diaphragm and intercostal muscles. **(M-S)**

▶ For every patient problem, there is a nursing diagnosis; for every nursing diagnosis, there is an outcome; for every outcome, there are interventions designed to make the outcome a reality. The key to answering NCLEX questions correctly is identifying the problem presented, formulating an outcome for that specific problem, and then selecting the intervention that will enable the patient to reach that specific outcome. **(FND)**

▶ Signs of meningeal irritation as seen in meningitis include nuchal rigidity, positive Brudzinski's sign, and a positive Kernig's sign. **(M-S)**

▶ Laboratory values indicating bacterial pneumomeningitis include elevated cerebrospinal fluid protein (above 100 mg/dl), decreased cerebrospinal fluid glucose (below 40 mg/dl), and increased white blood cell count (100 to 10,000/μl). **(M-S)**

▶ To promote rest in the very young child in a hospital setting, the first nursing action is to decrease environmental stimulation. **(PED)**

▶ To promote sleep in the very young child in a hospital setting, the nurse should ask the parents about the child's sleep rituals. **(PED)**

▶ Before magnetic resonance imaging, the patient should remove all objects containing metal, such as watches, bras, and jewelry. **(M-S)**

▶ Normally, food and medicine aren't restricted before magnetic resonance imaging. **(M-S)**

▶ The patient undergoing magnetic resonance imaging will lie supine on a padded table that will move through an imager. **(M-S)**

▶ The patient undergoing magnetic resonance imaging should be informed that he can ask questions during the procedure; however, he may be asked to lie still at certain times. **(M-S)**

▶ If a contrast medium is used during magnetic resonance imaging, advise the patient that he may experience diuresis when the medium is flushed from his body. **(M-S)**

▶ Hepatitis C is spread primarily through blood (posttransfusion or in people working with blood products), personal contact and, possibly, the fecal-oral route. **(M-S)**

▶ The best wound soak for an open, infected, draining wound is a hot-moist dressing. **(M-S)**

▶ The confirmation test for tuberculosis is a sputum culture. **(M-S)**

▶ Decadron (dexamethasone) is a steroidal anti-inflammatory drug used in the treatment of adrenal insufficiency. **(M-S)**

▶ During the first 24 hours following amputation, the residual limb is elevated on a pillow; after that time, the limb is placed flat to reduce the risk of hip flexion contracture. **(M-S)**

▶ A tourniquet should be in plain view at the bedside of the patient with an amputation. **(M-S)**

▶ An emergency tracheostomy set should be kept at the bedside of the patient suspected of having epiglottiditis. **(M-S)**

► The key word to use when reporting suspected cases of child abuse to the appropriate authorities is that child abuse is "suspected." **(PED)**

► The patient with acquired immunodeficiency syndrome shouldn't share a razor or toothbrush; however, there are no special precautions regarding dinnerware or laundry services. **(M-S)**

► Estriol level is used to assess fetal well-being, maternal renal functioning, and pregnancies complicated by diabetes. **(MAT)**

► Water accumulating in a ventilator tube should be removed. **(M-S)**

► A symptom of sensory overload is a feeling of distress and hyperarousal with impaired thinking and concentration. **(PSY)**

► *Sensory deprivation* refers to a state in which overall sensory input is decreased. **(PSY)**

► Sensory deprivation is manifested by daydreaming, inactivity, sleeping excessively, and reminiscing. **(PSY)**

► After total knee replacement surgery, the patient's knee is kept in maximum extension for 3 days. **(M-S)**

► Sjögren's syndrome is a chronic inflammatory disorder associated with a decrease in salivation and lacrimation; clinical manifestations include a dry mouth, dry eyes, and a dry vagina in a female. **(M-S)**

► The three brain barriers are the blood-brain barrier, blood-cerebrospinal fluid barrier, and brain-cerebrospinal fluid barrier. **(M-S)**

► Normal ranges and values of cerebrospinal fluid include protein: 15 to 45 mg/100 ml, glucose: (fasting) 50 to 75 mg/100 ml, red blood cells: 0, white blood cells: 0 to 4/µl, pH: 7.3, and potassium ions: 2.9 mmol/L. **(M-S)**

► To determine whether a cranial nerve is a motor nerve, use the following mnemonic:

I	II	III	IV	V	VI	VII	VIII	IX	X	XI	XII

Some Say Marry Money, But My Brother Says Bad Business Marry Money.

Here's how to interpret the above mnemonic: If the word begins with an S, it indicates a sensory nerve; if it starts with an M, it indicates a motor nerve; if it starts with a B, it indicates both a sensory and a motor nerve. **(M-S)**

▶ The Glasgow Coma Scale, on which the patient can obtain a score of 3 to 15, is used to evaluate the patient's level of consciousness, pupil reaction, and motor activity. **(M-S)**

▶ In homonymous hemianopsia, a condition of defective vision, the patient sees only half of the same visual field of each eye; therefore, he sees one half of normal vision. **(M-S)**

▶ Passive range-of-motion exercises are normally started 24 hours after a stroke and are performed four times a day. **(M-S)**

▶ The medical management goal in treating the patient with a transient ischemic attack is to prevent a cerebrovascular accident; therefore, the patient is given antihypertensive drugs, antiplatelet drugs or aspirin and, in some cases, warfarin sodium (Coumadin). **(M-S)**

▶ The patient with an intraperitoneal shunt should be observed for increased abdominal girth. **(M-S)**

▶ In determining acid-base problems, first note the pH. If it's above 7.45, it's a problem of acidosis; if it's below 7.35, it's a problem of alkalosis. Next, look at the partial pressure of arterial carbon dioxide ($Paco_2$). This is the respiratory indicator. If the pH is acidic and the $Paco_2$ is acidic (above 45 mm Hg), there's a match. The source of the problem, then, is respiration and is called respiratory acidosis. If the pH is alkaline and the $Paco_2$ is also alkaline (below 35 mm Hg), there's a match. The source of the problem, then, is respiration and is called respiratory alkalosis. If the $Paco_2$ is normal, look at the bicarbonate (HCO_3^-), which is the metabolic indicator, and note whether it's acidic (less than 22 mEq/L) or alkaline (greater than 26 mEq/L). See which value the pH matches to determine whether it's metabolic acidosis or metabolic alkalosis. If both the $Paco_2$ and HCO_3^- are abnormal, the body is compensating. If the pH has returned to normal and the $Paco_2$ or HCO_3^- is still normal, the body is in full compensation. **(M-S)**

▶ The Tensilon (edrophonium) test is used to confirm myasthenia gravis. **(M-S)**

▶ A masklike facial expression is a sign of myasthenia gravis and Parkinson's disease. **(M-S)**

▶ A sign of Paget's disease is bowleggedness. **(M-S)**

▶ For the patient abiding by Jewish custom, milk and meat shouldn't be served in the same meal. **(FND)**

▶ Don't permit smoking, use an aerosol spray, or shake bedsheets around a patient with a tracheostomy. **(M-S)**

▶ The best way to prevent disuse osteoporosis is to ambulate the patient. **(M-S)**

▶ Treatment for bleeding esophageal varices includes vasopressin, esophageal tamponade, iced saline lavage, and vitamin K.   **(M-S)**

▶ Pheochromocytoma is a catecholamine-secreting neoplasm of the adrenal medulla that results in an excessive production of epinephrine and norepinephrine.   **(M-S)**

▶ Clinical manifestations of pheochromocytoma include visual disturbance, headaches, hypertension, and elevated blood glucose levels; patients with this condition should avoid products containing caffeine.   **(M-S)**

▶ The patient shouldn't consume products containing caffeine, such as cola, coffee, or tea, for at least 8 hours before obtaining a 24-hour urine sample for vanillylmandelic acid.   **(M-S)**

▶ The best method for debriding a wound is to use a wet to dry dressing; remove the dressing once it has dried.   **(M-S)**

▶ The patient with an above-the-knee amputation should be placed in a prone position twice a day to prevent hip flexion contractures.   **(M-S)**

▶ The nurse shouldn't put anything, including a thermometer, in the mouth of the child who is suspected of having epiglottiditis.   **(M-S)**

▶ Signs of hip dislocation are one limb shorter than the other and an externally rotated limb.   **(M-S)**

▶ Extrapyramidal syndrome in the patient with Parkinson's disease is most likely caused by a deficiency of dopamine in the substantia nigra of the brain.   **(M-S)**

▶ Immediate care of a full-thickness skin graft in the patient with burns includes covering the site with a bulky dressing.   **(M-S)**

▶ The donor site of a skin graft should be left exposed to the air. **(M-S)**

▶ Any leaking around a T tube should be reported immediately to the doctor.   **(M-S)**

▶ Diphtheria is characterized by a pseudomembranous patch covering the posterior pharynx.   **(M-S)**

▶ A sign of tinea capitis in the child is a scratch on the scalp.   **(PED)**

▶ Kwell shampoo for head lice has been effective if there are no lice in the hair and there are no eggs (nits) attached to hair shafts.   **(M-S)**

▶ In the patient with a Steinmann pin in the femur, adverse signs include erythema, edema, and pain around the pin site. **(M-S)**

▶ Signs of chronic glaucoma include halos around lights, gradual loss of peripheral vision, and cloudiness of vision. **(M-S)**

▶ The patient with a transectional injury of C3 will need positive ventilation. **(M-S)**

▶ The nurse should keep the sac of myelomeningocele moist with normal saline solution. **(MAT)**

▶ After supratentorial surgery, the patient should be placed in semi-Fowler's position. **(M-S)**

▶ Frequent swallowing in a child after a tonsillectomy or an adenoidectomy may indicate excessive bleeding or hemorrhage. **(PED)**

▶ Generally, women with diabetes mellitus tend to have varying levels of hyperglycemia and have large but physically immature infants. **(MAT)**

▶ Compared with preoperative findings, the stress of surgery and anesthesia may cause a slight decrease in blood pressure and temperature and a slight increase in respiration. **(M-S)**

Index